Dr. Dvir Levin | THE RIGHT TO A FREE MIND

THE RIGHT TO A FREE MIND

Self-published - Dr. Dvir Levin
Content editing, language editing, proofreading, typesetting, and production: Dr. Dvir Levin

English edition | 2026
ISBN for the English edition: 978-965-93397-4-7

THE RIGHT TO A FREE MIND

From Coercion to Autonomy

The Evolution of Mental Health Rights in Israel and Worldwide

Dr. Dvir Levin

First Edition | August 2026

Author's Note and the Language of This Boo

This book addresses a field in which words themselves carry a history. Terms such as "madman," "mentally ill person," "insane," and "lunatic asylum" appeared for generations in medical, legal, and public discourse, and some still survive in the titles of older statutes, historical judgments, and official documents.

In this book, such terms are used only when they are necessary to understand a historical or legal source. In ordinary discussion, preference is given to expressions such as "a person living with a mental health condition," "a person experiencing mental distress," "patient," or other wording appropriate to the context.

This choice is not merely stylistic. One of the book's central arguments is that the transition from a model of coercion to a model of autonomy does not occur only in statutes and procedures; it also occurs in the way society describes the person. When the diagnosis replaces the person, it becomes easier to justify the loss of liberty. When the person remains at the center - with wishes, relationships, a history, rights, and the ability to participate in decisions - the starting point of care changes as well.

This book is not a substitute for individualized medical or legal advice. Its purpose is to analyze the historical, legal, and social development of the rights of people with mental health conditions, to compare different models, and to offer a framework for thinking about the proper balance among care, protection, liberty, and autonomy.

Contents

Contents - continued

Contents - continued

Introduction - Who Decides What Is Best for a Person?

Imagine an ordinary night in an ordinary apartment. A young man who has not slept for several nights walks from room to room, convinced that someone outside is watching him. His mother tries to speak with him, his father wonders whether to call for help, and he asks only to be left alone. An hour earlier he was still at home, surrounded by familiar objects and by people who know the story of his life. Within a short time, he may find himself facing a team he does not know, in an unfamiliar place, where the question of whether he can return home no longer depends on his wishes alone.

From one perspective, this is a story about saving a life. If the crisis escalates and he harms himself or someone else, everyone who was there will ask why no one intervened in time. From another perspective, it is a story about liberty. If it later becomes clear that there was no substantial danger, or that help could have been provided in another way, the very fact of being taken by force and kept behind a locked door will remain an event that cannot easily be undone. Both stories can be true at the same time.

That is why mental health is one of the places where abstract principles quickly become matters of body, door, key, and time. Words such as autonomy, proportionality, and dignity sound legal until the moment a person asks to leave and the door does not open. Words such as responsibility, protection, and dangerousness sound paternalistic until a family member tells the team: "If you discharge him now, I am genuinely afraid he will not survive the night." This book is written in the space between those two statements.

It does not set out to prove in advance that psychiatry oppressed or that psychiatry saved. Either claim on its own is too narrow. Psychiatry has saved people, relieved suffering, and returned many to life in the community; it has also operated, at different times, through institutions and practices that restricted liberty to an extent that is difficult to accept today. Law protected people from arbitrariness; for many years it also supplied a legal framework for coercion. Families were a source of protection and love; at times they were also part of a mechanism that made decisions in place of the person. History becomes most instructive when we stop choosing one side in advance and try to understand how all these forces worked together.

Few fields of medicine make the question "Who decides?" as charged as mental health. In most areas of modern medicine, the starting point is relatively clear: an adult with decision-making capacity may accept treatment, refuse it, seek a second opinion, leave a medical institution, and even prefer a choice that the treating team regards as less than optimal. The principle of informed consent reflects recognition that the patient's body and life belong first and foremost to the patient. Psychiatry, by contrast, stands at the point where the very capacity to choose may itself become part of the clinical discussion.

A person in an acute psychotic crisis may be convinced that family members are trying to poison him. A person in profound depression may say that she does not want to continue living. A person in a manic state may refuse all treatment, spend very large sums of money, and act in ways that he himself would not choose during a stable period. In such cases, the question whether to respect the choice cannot be separated from the question whether the choice expresses the person's wishes, the effects of the illness, or a complex combination of both. From this emerges one of the hardest dilemmas in a liberal democracy: when, if ever, may the state deprive a person of liberty in the name of protecting that person or others?

The dilemma is not new. For centuries, people whose behavior was viewed as unusual, incomprehensible, or dangerous were removed from the community. Some were imprisoned, some were held in religious institutions or asylums, and some lived at society's margins without treatment. With the development of psychiatry in the eighteenth and nineteenth centuries, an important change occurred: what had once been understood as sin, madness, or moral deviance increasingly came to be understood as illness deserving treatment. Yet that humanistic revolution contained a paradox. Recognizing the person as ill rather than criminal opened the door to treatment - but also granted medicine broad authority to decide on the person's behalf.

This is how the modern psychiatric institution emerged: a place explicitly intended to heal and protect, but also a place of separation, discipline, and deprivation of liberty. During the nineteenth and twentieth centuries, the assumption became established that a person's best interests might justify hospitalization even without consent. Courts and legislatures developed doctrines that allowed the state to act both through its responsibility toward those deemed unable to protect themselves and through its duty to protect the public. In American legal terminology, these rationales came to be described, among other things, as parens patriae - the state's protective role - and the police power - its authority to preserve public order and safety.

During the twentieth century, however, the picture began to change. Harsh experiences in closed institutions, criticism of hospitalization conditions, the development of psychiatric medications, civil-rights movements, and the strengthening constitutional language of liberty and dignity produced a profound shift. In the United States, the Supreme Court held in O'Connor v. Donaldson (1975) that mental illness alone does not justify the prolonged confinement of a person who is not dangerous and can live safely in the community. Four years later, Addington v. Texas raised the evidentiary standard required for involuntary civil commitment. In Europe, the European Court of Human Rights held in Winterwerp v. the Netherlands (1979) that deprivation of liberty on the ground of mental disorder must satisfy basic conditions, including objective medical evidence and an ongoing relationship between the disorder and the justification for confinement.

At the same time, a broad process of deinstitutionalization began - the reduction of large psychiatric hospitals and the development of community-based services. The process was neither uniform nor consistently successful. Where beds were closed without an adequate community system being built, the result was sometimes a shift from psychiatric institutions to homelessness, prisons, or repeated cycles of hospitalization. A central lesson follows and will accompany the book throughout: rights are not realized merely by prohibiting coercion. A person does not become free simply because the hospital door opens if there is no housing, treatment, income, social connection, or support that makes life in the community possible.

Israel's mental-health system developed within this tension. The Treatment of Mentally Ill Persons Law, 1955, was one of the state's early statutes in this field and largely reflected the outlook of its time: broad professional authority, institutional care, and oversight that appears limited from a contemporary perspective. In 1991 it was replaced by the Mental Health Treatment Law, 1991, which reorganized involuntary examination and hospitalization, the powers of district psychiatrists, psychiatric committees, and mechanisms for reviewing decisions. The new law was a significant step, but it was enacted just before a series of constitutional and social changes transformed the language of rights in Israel.

A year later, Basic Law: Human Dignity and Liberty was enacted. In 1996, the Patient's Rights Law established, among other things, a statutory framework for dignity, privacy, and informed consent. In 1998, the Equal Rights for Persons with Disabilities Law was enacted. In 2000, the Community Rehabilitation of Persons with Mental Disabilities Law - renamed in 2024 as the Community Rehabilitation of Persons Coping with Mental Health Conditions Law - gave community rehabilitation an independent statutory status. Amendment 18 to the Legal Capacity and Guardianship Law, adopted in 2016, advanced alternatives to guardianship in Israel, including supported decision-making. Each of these developments changed the context in which the 1991 law must be read, even though that law remains in force and has been amended over time.

International law changed as well. The United Nations Convention on the Rights of Persons with Disabilities (CRPD), adopted in 2006, placed autonomy, equal recognition before the law, and life in the community at the center of the discussion. The CRPD Committee has interpreted its provisions in a manner that is particularly critical of deprivation of liberty and involuntary treatment based on disability. In 2023, the World Health Organization and the Office of the United Nations High Commissioner for Human Rights issued joint guidance on mental-health legislation, calling on states to ground their laws in human rights, consent, and community-based services, and to reduce reliance on coercion very substantially.

The difference between the two worldviews is clear. The traditional approach asks: when may treatment be imposed in order to prevent danger or deterioration? The newer approach adds a prior question: what conditions, services, and forms of support could have been provided before coercion came to appear unavoidable? It asks us to examine not only the moment when a ward door is locked, but everything that preceded it - access to care, trust, housing, continuity of treatment, the ability to make decisions with support, home-based care, crisis houses, and the participation of people with lived experience in designing services.

The book is therefore structured as both a chronological and conceptual movement. It begins in periods when people experiencing mental disorders were at times viewed as threats, sinners, or people to be removed. It continues through the birth of psychiatry and the institution, the institutionalization of coercion, and the legal legitimization of deprivation of liberty. From there it moves to criticism, deinstitutionalization, human rights, the development of Israeli legislation, and the emergence of recovery and rehabilitation models. Only once that path is understood can we return to the hard questions of the twenty-first century: Is involuntary hospitalization still justified? What should the threshold of dangerousness be? May a person refuse medication when judgment is impaired? Can restraint ever be considered a therapeutic measure? Is psychiatry with less coercion practically possible - perhaps, in the future, with almost none?

The book offers no single simple answer. A position that treats every form of coercion as an absolute wrong ignores situations in which a person faces an immediate and serious danger and is unable to accept help. A position that treats coercion as an ordinary therapeutic tool ignores the extraordinary power involved in depriving a person of liberty and the risk that an exception will become routine. The real challenge is to build a system capable of protecting life without erasing the person whose life it seeks to protect; a system that recognizes that even during a severe crisis, a person does not cease to be a rights-holder.

This is the book's starting point: mental health is not only a field of medicine. It is a test of the limits of state power, the professional authority of the physician, the responsibility of the family, the duty of the community, and the meaning we give to dignity, liberty, and autonomy precisely at the moment when it is easiest to argue that someone else knows best.

PART ONE

BEFORE THERE WERE RIGHTS

THE BIRTH OF INSTITUTIONAL PSYCHIATRY

Chapter One

From Madness to Mental Illness

Before Psychiatry

There is no single point in time at which mental illness was "invented." Throughout history, people have experienced anxiety, depression, confusion, manic behavior, hallucinations, delusions, and other phenomena that we would now describe in psychiatric language. What changed fundamentally was the way society interpreted those experiences and the person who experienced them.

In ancient societies, psychological disturbances were sometimes attributed to supernatural forces, spirits, curses, or religious punishment. Elsewhere, early bodily explanations also existed. In the Greek world, attempts can already be found to understand mental states as part of the body's functioning rather than exclusively as the result of divine intervention. For centuries, however, religious, moral, medical, and social explanations existed side by side. There was no "psychiatry" in the modern sense, and no single profession possessed authority to define what constituted mental disorder or what treatment was appropriate.

Society's treatment of people whose behavior was regarded as unusual was not uniform either. Some lived within families and communities; others were kept in shelters, poorhouses, religious institutions, or prisons. The history of mental-health care is therefore not a simple story of a transition from barbarity to progress. There were periods in which community arrangements allowed relatively flexible forms of life, and reforms undertaken in the name of humanity that ultimately led to the expansion of closed institutions. Already at this stage a paradox appears that will recur throughout the book: an action intended to protect a person can also create a new system for controlling that person.

The shift toward medical thinking was profound. When unusual behavior is explained as sin or moral defect, the natural response may be punishment, shame, or exclusion. When the same behavior is explained as illness, the possibility of treatment opens. This was an enormous humanistic achievement, but it carried a possible cost: if the illness is understood as impairing judgment, the physician may acquire authority to decide what is best for the patient even against the patient's wishes.

In the eighteenth and early nineteenth centuries, movements developed in Europe that later became associated with "moral treatment." In France, the movement is identified with Philippe Pinel and Jean-Baptiste Pussin; in England, with William Tuke and the York Retreat. The word "moral" here does not refer to moralism in the modern sense, but to an approach that sought to replace violent measures and harsh bodily treatment with an orderly environment, more humane relations, routine, work, conversation, and supervision. Historical scholarship shows that this approach was more complex than the familiar symbolic story of "freeing the insane from their chains." It did contain humanistic elements, but it remained largely institutional, with staff determining the boundaries of patients' lives.

Romanticization should be avoided. Restraints remained in use in many institutions, and some methods of treatment harmed the body and dignity. Even so, the very idea that a person experiencing mental disorder deserved systematic attention, treatment, and a measure of dignity - rather than mere exclusion - was a decisive step toward the emergence of modern psychiatry.

When a medical field develops, it does not merely offer treatment; it also creates categories. Diagnoses give names to phenomena and enable research, professional communication, and treatment planning. At the same time, they can become social identities. A person is no longer simply someone who hears voices; he or she becomes a particular kind of "patient." Society may then view that person as unpredictable, irresponsible, or dangerous even when there is no individual basis for doing so.

In mental health, the consequences of labeling were especially serious because diagnosis was for many years closely tied to questions of legal and practical capacity. If the physician believes that a person does not understand the condition, it becomes easier to conclude that the person's wishes should not carry full weight. From there it is a short step to paternalism: the assumption that the professional may choose for the patient because the professional knows better what is required.

Paternalism does not necessarily arise from indifference or cruelty. Sometimes it grows precisely from genuine concern. A physician who sees a person endangering himself may feel that non-intervention would amount to abandonment. A family fearing suicide may regard involuntary hospitalization as a life-saving measure. The problem begins when concern becomes a source of almost unlimited authority, when there is no mechanism of review, and when the assumption of incapacity is applied to an entire group rather than examined in relation to a specific decision and a specific person.

One of the deepest associations in the history of psychiatry is the connection between mental illness and dangerousness. Even today, there are circumstances in which an acute mental disorder may be associated with a genuine risk. History, however, shows that the public conception of dangerousness was far broader than the empirical risk. Unpredictable behavior, unusual speech, or deviation from social norms were often treated as threats in themselves.

Two different questions therefore became entangled: whether the person needed treatment, and whether society wanted to remove the person. A psychiatric institution could serve a therapeutic purpose and a public-order purpose at the same time. This merger would later stand at the heart of legal debates over involuntary hospitalization: does the state deprive a person of liberty in order to treat, in order to protect the public, or because it has no other framework for responding to acute distress?

The question is not merely historical. When a mental-health system lacks housing solutions, home-based treatment, or crisis alternatives, the hospital may once again become the place into which social problems that are not purely medical are channeled. This is why it is so important to distinguish diagnosis from dangerousness, need for treatment from justification for deprivation of liberty, and medical responsibility from social responsibility.

The Moment Medicine Acquires Power

The development of psychiatry shifted the center of authority. In place of the priest, judge, or community leader, the physician gradually appeared as the expert. That expertise made more advanced diagnosis and treatment possible, but it also gave medical language legal force. A determination that a person was "ill" began to affect the possibility of hospitalization, management of property, status within the family, and at times civil liberty itself.

In this sense, the history of the rights of people with mental health conditions is also the history of an effort to place limits on expertise. Not because psychiatric knowledge should be rejected, but because medical expertise is not the same as unlimited moral or legal authority. A physician can assess a mental state; whether that assessment may justify deprivation of liberty is already a question of law, rights, and proportionality.

From the person's own perspective, the change in language was not merely semantic. Someone who had been regarded within the community as cursed, sinful, weak-willed, or dangerous could, within the new medical framework, be understood as experiencing a condition that could be observed, described, and treated. This was real human progress. The ability to say that psychological suffering is not evidence of moral failure opened the way to a different kind of compassion, to reduced blame, and to a search for treatment rather than punishment. Yet the same development created a new professional category: the psychiatric patient. As medical knowledge expanded, so did the power of those authorized to determine who was ill, what behavior was abnormal, and when intervention was required.

Here begins one of the paradoxes that will accompany the book throughout. Recognizing suffering as a medical problem can free a person from blame, but it can also transfer part of the authority over that person's life to experts. It can enable treatment while also justifying supervision. It can protect against ridicule and punishment while creating a label that follows a person long after the crisis has passed. The history of mental health is therefore not a straight movement from darkness to light. It is a process in which every advance opened new possibilities and new questions about the limits of power.

It is also important to remember that most people who experienced psychological distress throughout history did not live in institutions. They lived in families, streets, villages, and communities; some were supported and others were hidden away. The family was the primary caregiver long before the state assumed responsibility. This created deep dependence on personal relationships and local resources. A person surrounded by a family with means could receive a very different kind of protection from someone left alone. The birth of institutional psychiatry was therefore also a response to this inequality: an attempt to create a public framework in place of care that depended almost entirely on the generosity, capacity, and patience of relatives.

The move from community to institution changed not only the place of care but the identity of the decision-maker. At home, even when the family was paternalistic, life unfolded within a familiar relationship. In the institution, the daily routine was set by a system. This is the point at which the question of treatment begins to become a question of governance: who opens the door, who determines when people get up, who decides whether a person may leave, and who has authority to say that the person's resistance is itself a symptom of illness.

The transition from the language of "madness" to the language of medical diagnosis also changed a person's biography. Once an experience receives a professional name, it becomes documentable, researchable, and treatable, but it also enters a record that may accompany the person. A name can bring relief: it can show that the experience is known and that others have lived through it. It can also become a burden when society reads the person through the diagnosis rather than reading the person's life.

This tension does not belong only to the modern era. From psychiatry's beginnings, it became clear that the words used to describe distress create a framework of possibilities: who is authorized to speak, who is treated as credible, and who may decide what is normal and what is deviant.

The very idea of "illness" carried a double promise. On one hand, it weakened the view that unusual behavior was sin, moral failure, or a defect of character. A person who suffers is not necessarily to blame for that suffering. On the other hand, when the medical explanation becomes exclusive, it may conceal the context in which distress arose: poverty, violence, loss, loneliness, war, or family relationships. Psychiatry gradually learned that the mind exists neither only inside the brain nor only inside society; it takes shape in the encounter between them.

This is why the historical perspective matters. It reminds us that diagnoses, institutions, and treatment methods do not fall from the sky. They are created in a particular period, from particular knowledge and particular values. That knowledge does not invalidate science. It requires humility: what seems self-evident today may look partial in the future, just as some explanations of the past now seem foreign to us.

The next chapter turns to the place where this power took physical form: the asylum and the psychiatric institution. There, for the first time, a complete system developed in which treatment, residence, work, supervision, and discipline existed under one roof - and sometimes behind the same locked door.

Chapter Two

The Rise of Asylums and Psychiatric Institutions

An Institution Born as a Promise

It is easy to look back at the nineteenth-century psychiatric hospital and see it primarily as a symbol of oppression. Yet to understand why the institutional model expanded so rapidly, it is important to remember that it was initially presented as a humanitarian reform. Instead of leaving people in severe psychological distress in prisons, poorhouses, or family settings unable to provide care, reformers proposed a dedicated place in which they could receive protection, order, and treatment.

Many institutions were established outside cities, in surroundings regarded as quiet and healthful. The underlying belief was that removing a person from the environment in which the illness had emerged, and providing routine, work, rest, and moderate discipline, could promote recovery. The 'moral treatment' associated with Pinel, Pussin, and Tuke influenced this model. In the United States as well, a nineteenth-century movement developed to establish public asylums, and Dorothea Dix later campaigned for greater public responsibility toward people with mental illness.

The promise was twofold: humanity and treatment. Yet in many places the very success of the idea produced a new problem. As the number of patients grew, institutions intended to be small and therapeutic became enormous systems. When staffing did not increase accordingly and stays became longer, therapeutic routine turned into administrative regime. The institution was no longer simply a place where a person received treatment; it became the world in which that person lived.

Life in a large institution meant that the boundaries between treatment and private life almost disappeared. Waking and sleeping hours, meals, movement, clothing, visits, and work were determined by the framework. Even when each individual decision seemed reasonable from the standpoint of institutional management, their accumulation created profound dependence.

The sociologist Erving Goffman later described psychiatric hospitals as part of the category of 'total institutions' - settings in which large groups of people live and conduct their activities under a single authority, with the main spheres of life taking place in the same location and within the same system. The concept was critical, but it helped clarify how an institution can alter a person's identity even without direct violence. As everyday choices are reduced, a person may gradually lose skills, initiative, and a sense of ownership over life.

Later scholarship also used the term 'institutionalization' to describe adaptation to the system itself: a person learns what is expected in order to receive privileges, what should not be asked, when it is better to remain silent, and when compliance is rewarded. Behavior that may appear from the outside as a 'lack of motivation' can sometimes be the result of years in which independent choice was rarely required.

The boundary between treatment and discipline was one of the points at which the institutional model became problematic. Routine, activity, and occupation can have therapeutic value. When imposed, however, they may become instruments of control. Even the idea of a calm and orderly environment can be used to justify broad restrictions on movement, contact with family members, and personal belongings.

Within an institution, a patient's resistance can easily be interpreted as a symptom. If a person complains about conditions, is that legitimate criticism or a sign of 'lack of insight'? If the person asks to leave, is that a choice that should be respected or evidence that the person does not understand the condition? This is a structural problem: when the same authority is responsible both for diagnosis and for controlling the environment, it is difficult to create a space in which disagreement is not immediately medicalized.

One of the central lessons of modern mental-health law follows from this problem: a decision to deprive a person of liberty cannot remain an internal clinical matter alone. It requires legal conditions, external review, a right to be heard, and a route of appeal. These safeguards were not present from the outset; they developed after decades in which psychiatric hospitalization rested largely on professional and family discretion.

The psychiatric institution also served a social function. It provided a place for people who could not live without support in the community, while the community itself offered very little support. Poor families, families without resources, or families exhausted by prolonged crises could not always cope. In the absence of supported housing, day services, or home-based treatment, hospitalization was sometimes the only available option.

A cycle therefore emerged: because the institution was the principal solution, resources were invested in it; and because resources were invested there, alternatives failed to develop. When a person remained hospitalized for years, community ties weakened, the possibility of employment diminished, and returning to life outside the institution became more difficult. The system created part of the dependence that was later used to justify continued hospitalization.

This is an important distinction between illness and social disability. A person may need medical treatment, but the duration of institutionalization may be shaped not only by the severity of illness, but also by the absence of a home, income, employment, relationships, and community services. The rehabilitation approach that developed during the twentieth century would attempt to break this cycle through rights and services outside the hospital.

By the beginning of the twentieth century, large psychiatric hospitals were a central component of health systems in many countries. At the same time, new biological and psychological theories developed, but for many hospitalized people treatment options remained limited. Before the emergence of modern antipsychotic medications, institutions had to manage severe acute conditions with measures that today, in some cases, are regarded as harmful or unacceptable.

Overcrowding and pressure contributed in various places to declining quality of care. Institutions originally intended for recovery sometimes became settings for long-term custodial care. Out of this situation eventually emerged two movements that appear opposed but were in fact complementary: on one hand, a search for more effective medical treatments; on the other, a demand to protect the rights of hospitalized people even when intervention was undertaken in the name of medicine.

The Paradox of the Institution

The history of the psychiatric institution cannot be summarized simply in terms of good or bad. At times it was a genuine place of refuge for people rejected by society, and at other times a site of serious deprivation of liberty. It provided care during periods in which alternatives did not exist, yet it sometimes delayed their creation. It was born from a desire to separate mental illness from criminality, but it also created another form of civil confinement.

This paradox matters because it prevents a common error in contemporary debate. A move into the community does not itself guarantee rights, just as hospitalization does not necessarily preclude proper care. The central questions are what options are actually available to the person, how much power is concentrated in the system, and what mechanisms of oversight exist when the state restricts liberty.

To understand how an institution born as a humanitarian promise could become a restrictive environment, one must examine daily life rather than laws alone. A large institution needs routine: waking times, meals, medication rounds, physician visits, bathing, activities, and sleep. As the number of residents increases, adapting the routine to the individual becomes more difficult. Decisions that seem small - when smoking is allowed, where one may sit, whether a door may be closed, when a visitor may be received - become part of a system of control. This does not necessarily happen because anyone intends to humiliate; large organizations naturally tend to prefer order over exceptions.

This is an important difference between intention and outcome. An institution may be created from a sincere desire to protect and treat, while still producing a life in which a person has almost no opportunity to make decisions. When this continues for months and years, the loss is not limited to freedom of movement. A person may lose skills of choice, money management, cooking, work, social relationships, and even a sense of time. Release from such an institution is not comparable to leaving a brief hospitalization; it requires rebuilding a life that has become accustomed to being organized by instructions.

The architecture itself conveyed a message. A gate, a corridor, a locked ward, and the division between staff and patients are not merely technical details. They define who is inside and who is outside, who holds the key and who must ask permission. Some institutions also created open spaces, gardens, and workshops as part of a therapeutic vision; in others, crowding and separation intensified. Both tendencies sometimes existed side by side. The history of the institution therefore cannot be told only as a history of failure. It also provided shelter and treatment to people who, in some cases, had no other response available. The problem was that protection could easily become a framework that was difficult to leave.

This tension explains why the later debate over deinstitutionalization was never simple. Those who saw only the institutional gates wanted to open them; those who also knew the loneliness and poverty outside feared what would happen the day after discharge. A principle that will recur throughout this book is already visible here: genuine freedom is not merely the removal of a restriction. It requires conditions that make it possible to live outside that restriction.

To understand the power of the institution, it is also necessary to think about time. In a private home or community, a day consists of thousands of small decisions that are barely noticed: when to get up, what to eat, whom to speak with, whether to go outside, whether to close a door and be alone. In a large institution, many of those decisions are transferred to a shared schedule. Violence is not required to diminish autonomy; it can be enough that every small choice requires permission. The longer the stay, the more the structure becomes a world of its own.

From this developed the phenomenon later described as 'institutionalization': the person adapts to the framework until the ability to live outside it weakens. That adaptation is not evidence of personal weakness. It is a rational response to an environment in which initiative is not always needed and may at times even be discouraged. Someone who has not bought food, managed bills, planned a journey, or chosen how to spend the day for years needs more than a discharge order to return to independent life. Legal freedom may arrive in a single day; practical freedom is rebuilt slowly.

The paradox is that an institution can be restrictive and protective at the same time. For a person without a home, family, or income, its gates are not only a barrier that prevents exit; they may also be a wall protecting against hunger, loneliness, and violence outside. Criticism of the institution is therefore incomplete if it does not ask what awaits beyond the gate. Closing a bed does not necessarily open an opportunity. For a move into the community to amount to liberation rather than abandonment, the community must be a place that contains treatment, housing, relationships, and meaning.

The next chapter examines the point at which institution and treatment became not merely a framework but an explicit mechanism of coercion: hospitalization without consent, involuntary treatment, restraint and seclusion, and the way in which the concept of 'dangerousness' became the principal legal gateway to the deprivation of liberty.

Chapter Three

When Treatment and Confinement Become Coercion

What Is Psychiatric Coercion?

Coercion in mental health is not a single act. It is a continuum of interventions in which a person's wishes are restricted or replaced. At one end are informal pressures: a family member saying, 'If you do not take the medication, you cannot stay at home'; a clinician implying that refusal will lead to hospitalization; or a service making access conditional on compliance. At the other end are clear legal and physical measures: compulsory examination, involuntary hospitalization, medication without consent, mechanical restraint, seclusion, and restrictions on movement.

What these situations share is an imbalance of power. During psychiatric hospitalization, particularly in a locked ward, the person does not always have a practical ability to say 'no' and leave. Formal consent must therefore be examined carefully: was it given voluntarily, with understanding, and without a disproportionate threat? Modern law attempts to distinguish consensual treatment from coercive treatment, but reality is more complex than a simple binary division.

One of the oldest justifications for coercion is the assumption that the state may protect a person who, at that moment, is unable to protect himself or herself. In situations of acute suicidality, severe psychosis, or extreme confusion, immediate intervention may save a life. From this perspective, a person's refusal is not necessarily an expression of autonomous choice; it may result from a serious impairment of judgment.

The argument is especially strong in an emergency. If a person is about to jump from a bridge, society is not required to wait for a full judicial process before preventing the act. The difficulty begins when the logic of emergency is extended over long periods. Saving a life over a matter of minutes is not the same as depriving someone of liberty for weeks or months. The longer the intervention continues, the stronger the justification, reassessment, and independent review that are required.

Another central justification is dangerousness to others. Every state has both authority and responsibility to protect the public against serious and concrete danger. In mental health, however, there is a risk of conflating diagnosis with risk. Most people living with mental disorders are not violent, and the relationship between diagnosis and violence is influenced by many factors, including substance use, prior history, social circumstances, and treatment. A rights-based system therefore cannot accept the equation 'mental illness = dangerousness.' It must require an individualized assessment. Even where risk exists, one must ask how serious and immediate it is, whether a less restrictive alternative is available, and for how long the restriction can be justified.

During the twentieth century, 'dangerousness' became one of the main gateways to involuntary hospitalization because it creates a bridge between medicine and law. The psychiatrist assesses mental state and risk; the law determines when that assessment justifies deprivation of liberty. This bridge is not without difficulty. Risk assessment is never prophecy, and error is possible in both directions: releasing a person who is in genuine danger, or hospitalizing a person who would not have harmed himself, herself, or anyone else.

One of the most sensitive concepts is 'lack of insight' - a situation in which a person does not accept that he or she is ill, or disagrees with the diagnosis and the need for treatment. Clinically, lack of insight can be part of certain disorders. Legally, however, disagreement must not automatically be equated with incapacity.

A person can understand the information and still decide differently from the treating team. Autonomy includes, to some extent, the right to make decisions that others regard as unwise. In general medicine, we recognize that a competent person may refuse life-saving surgery for religious or personal reasons. The psychiatric question is when the disorder itself impairs the ability to understand, weigh, or communicate a decision to a degree that can justify intervention.

Modern law increasingly tends to assess decision-making capacity in relation to a particular decision rather than as a general status. A person may struggle with a complex treatment decision while still being able to choose where to live, whom to speak with, and what to eat. This approach later underpins supported decision-making: instead of asking only, 'Is the person capable?', the question becomes, 'What support would enable the person to decide for himself or herself?'

From Institutional Coercion to the Question of Limits

As psychiatry became part of the machinery of the state, coercion acquired a more formal structure. The decision to hospitalize was no longer merely a family or institutional act; it became a decision involving a physician, an authority, documents, and sometimes a court. In one sense this was progress: power that had previously been exercised vaguely received a legal source and rules. Yet formal regulation also made coercion a more familiar and routine part of the system.

Three questions that history often mixed together must be distinguished. The first is medical: what is the person's condition and what might help? The second concerns risk: what might happen if there is no intervention? The third is legal: who may restrict liberty, under what conditions, and for how long? A physician may be convinced that treatment would help and yet there may be no legal basis for coercion. Conversely, an emergency may justify a short restriction even before a complete diagnostic picture exists. Distinguishing these questions would become fundamental to the development of mental-health law.

From the person's perspective, the legal distinctions are not always visible during a crisis. The person encounters a door that will not open, a team asking him or her to remain, and sometimes family members who agree with the team. What appears to the system as a sequence of separate powers may be experienced as a single event of lost control. A discussion of coercion therefore cannot be limited to whether each stage was lawful. It must also examine how power was exercised: was it explained, was the person's voice heard, was a less restrictive option available, and was the justification reconsidered when the situation changed?

At this point, the central theme of this book comes into view. Psychiatric coercion is unusual within medicine not merely because physical force is sometimes used. It is unusual because professional knowledge and state power are joined within the same act. The individual is not only a patient receiving a recommendation; in certain situations, he or she is also a citizen whose liberty is restricted in the name of treatment or safety. This combination requires law to enter the treatment room - not to replace the physician, but to define the limits of power.

The judicial decisions and legal tests that began to limit this power are examined in Chapter Five. The distinction between hospitalization and treatment, and the particular questions raised by treatment without consent and physical restraint, are examined in Part Seven. For now, it is enough to understand how the question arose: once treatment ceases to be voluntary, who decides where protection ends and deprivation of liberty begins?

The history of psychiatric coercion is not a story in which 'coercion belonged to the past and no longer exists.' Involuntary hospitalization continues in advanced health systems. The principal change lies in the demand that it be justified. Instead of broad authority based on diagnosis alone, modern law requires legal criteria, dangerousness or serious need as defined by local law, proportionality, review, and a limited duration. At the same time, the contemporary disability-rights movement asks an even more fundamental question: whether the very structure of legislation based on psychosocial or mental disability is compatible with equality.

To understand how this debate developed, we must now move into the twentieth century - the period in which psychiatry became a medical specialty with powerful biological tools while the psychiatric institution reached the height of its authority. There the tension between the wish to heal and the capacity to control became still sharper.

Psychiatric coercion becomes especially clear in the moment of crisis. Imagine a person arriving at an emergency department after a sleepless night, agitated and convinced that someone is following him. His family is frightened, the staff is trying to determine whether there is danger, and he himself asks to leave. Within minutes a deep gap opens between perspectives. From his point of view, he is surrounded by people who do not believe him and want to control him; from the team's point of view, allowing him to leave may end in disaster; from the family's point of view, the very possibility that the system might discharge him feels like abandonment. Coercion does not necessarily begin when a door is locked. It begins when each side feels that there is no longer a shared language with the other.

In such situations it is easy, in retrospect, to speak of the correct decision. In real time, information is incomplete and risk is uncertain. No test provides a binary answer to whether a person will harm himself, herself, or someone else. Professionals act under time pressure, moral responsibility, and legal anxiety. Precisely for this reason, a rights-based system cannot rely on a general instruction to 'use professional judgment.' It must create a series of safeguards: assess the intensity of risk, ask what alternatives have been attempted, separate disagreement from incapacity, document the decision, and enable external review.

What happens after the crisis passes also matters. A person may remember for years the moment he was taken by force, the struggle in the corridor, or the feeling that no one listened. Even if the intervention prevented harm, it can leave a residue that shapes the next encounter with the healthcare system. Someone who experiences treatment as coercion may conceal symptoms in the future in order to avoid being placed in the same situation again. A paradox therefore emerges: an action intended to protect can make early treatment more difficult during the next crisis.

There is a reason why psychiatric coercion generates sharper controversy than many other medical restrictions. It often occurs precisely when there is disagreement about reality itself. A person experiencing persecutory thoughts may be convinced that the team is part of the threat from which he is trying to escape; the team, in turn, may interpret refusal of help as evidence that the crisis is deepening. The same act therefore receives two opposite meanings: to the team it is protection, while to the person it confirms the fear that someone is trying to control him.

In such a situation it is not enough to declare that one side is simply 'right.' Professionals may need to act even when there is no time to build full agreement, but the way in which they use power may determine the relationship after the crisis has passed. A person may later acknowledge that help was needed and still feel humiliated by the way it was delivered. A person may also continue to oppose the decision itself even when the system remains convinced that it prevented danger. Both experiences can exist without canceling each other out.

From this emerges an idea that will accompany us to the end of the book: the legitimacy of coercion is not determined only by whether there were grounds to intervene. It also depends on the degree of force used, the duration, the opportunity to appeal, the quality of explanation, and the effort to restore partnership as soon as possible. Coercion may be a brief event within care that otherwise respects the person, or it may become an entire language in which every disagreement is answered by authority. The difference is not semantic; it shapes whether the person emerges from the crisis with a sense of rescue, a sense of injury, or a complex mixture of both.

This is why preventing coercion must be understood broadly. It does not begin with the question of how to conduct involuntary hospitalization more respectfully, but with the question of what should have existed weeks and months earlier so that the crisis would be less likely to reach that point. Continuity with a clinician, the possibility of receiving help at home, an agreed crisis plan, a trusted person who knows how to respond, and services available outside conventional hours all belong to the story of coercion even though they do not look like legal mechanisms. Sometimes the best way to protect a person's rights at the extreme moment is to build a system that reduces the likelihood of reaching it.

PART TWO

THE ERA OF INSTITUTIONALIZED COERCION

Chapter Four

Psychiatry in the Twentieth Century: Between Hope and Power

A Medical Profession Searching for Tools

The twentieth century transformed psychiatry from the ground up. It was a period of genuine scientific progress, the creation of new treatments, and a gradual transition from custodial institutions toward a medicine that sought to intervene actively. Yet it was also a period in which the desire to treat quickly, in the face of profound suffering and limited alternatives, led to extensive use of interventions that later became symbols of the dangers of medical power.

At the beginning of the century, many people hospitalized in psychiatric institutions had no effective biological treatment in the sense familiar today. Staff relied on the institutional environment, routine, work, calming measures, psychotherapy where available, and at times a range of physical interventions. People with severe psychosis, profound depression, or catatonic states could remain in institutions for years. Medicine did not operate in a vacuum: it confronted people in real distress, families with few options, and institutions that were becoming increasingly overcrowded.

This context is essential for understanding the enthusiasm with which new treatments were received in the 1930s and 1940s. Insulin therapy, chemically induced convulsions, electroconvulsive therapy, and psychosurgery emerged in a period when options were limited. Some of these treatments were later abandoned; others changed profoundly. ECT, the most prominent example, remains an accepted medical treatment for certain conditions today. History does not justify uncontrolled use, but it explains why professionals sometimes viewed difficult interventions as hope rather than cruelty.

Electroconvulsive therapy was developed in Italy in 1938 by Ugo Cerletti and Lucio Bini. In its early period it was administered under conditions very different from contemporary practice. Over time, anesthesia, muscle relaxation, monitoring, and more precise protocols were introduced. The fact that ECT survived while other treatments were abandoned underscores the importance of distinguishing criticism of historical methods of use from contemporary evaluation of efficacy and safety.

For the purposes of this book, ECT illustrates a broader dilemma: a treatment can be effective and still raise difficult questions of consent. In severe depression, catatonia, or life-threatening circumstances, physicians may regard it as essential; the patient may fear it, oppose it, or be in a state in which decision-making capacity is in question. The discussion therefore cannot end with 'Is the treatment good?' It must also ask: 'Who decided?', 'Under what conditions?', 'What alternatives were considered?', and 'How was the person's own preference weighed?'

The history of ECT also demonstrates the power of cultural images. Films, literature, and accounts of involuntary use created a public memory of treatment done to a person rather than with the person. Even when the technology changed, the memory remained. A system that seeks trust cannot be satisfied with saying that the treatment is safer; it must acknowledge the history, explain, involve the person, and preserve choice to the greatest extent possible.

Psychosurgery: When Hope Outpaced the Evidence

In 1935, the Portuguese neurologist Egas Moniz proposed the prefrontal leucotomy. In the years that followed, psychosurgery spread, particularly in the United States, where variations of lobotomy were offered to people with a range of psychiatric conditions. The history of the field reflects a combination of therapeutic desperation, professional enthusiasm, early outcomes that appeared promising, institutional pressure, and the absence of research and ethical standards comparable to those accepted today.

Some patients experienced serious changes in personality, functioning, and cognition. With the emergence of antipsychotic medications, increasing public criticism, and a better understanding of harms, lobotomy declined. Modern psychosurgery, when performed, is fundamentally different in precision, indication, and oversight; nevertheless, this historical chapter remains a warning about situations in which professional authority, scarcity of alternatives, and faith in a new intervention substitute for long-term evidence and meaningful consent.

The lesson is broader than psychosurgery. In any system in which the patient depends on the professional and the institution, medical innovation requires especially strong safeguards. When the person does not have full freedom to refuse, scientific uncertainty acquires an additional moral and legal dimension.

In the early 1950s, chlorpromazine entered psychiatric use and marked the beginning of the psychopharmacological revolution. For the first time, psychotic symptoms could be reduced in some patients to a degree that allowed greater functioning and more sustained discharge from the institution. Additional medications later appeared for depression, anxiety, bipolar disorder, and other conditions.

Medication had an enormous impact on the possibility of community-based treatment. Yet another paradox emerged. The tool that enabled many people to leave institutions also became, at times, a central instrument of coercion both inside and outside them. Medication is not neutral: it may provide substantial relief, but it may also cause adverse effects and influence alertness, movement, weight, sexual functioning, and subjective experience. If the person is not a partner in choosing the medication, dosage, and balance between effectiveness and adverse effects, medical treatment may be experienced as control.

The development of psychopharmacology therefore did not eliminate the question of rights; it changed its form. In addition to the closed institution, community life became possible - but so too did the extension of therapeutic supervision into the community through orders, monitoring, or conditions attached to services.

From the Passive Patient to the Question of Partnership

During the first half of the twentieth century, the medical relationship was generally paternalistic. The physician decided, and the patient was expected to trust the physician. This was not unique to psychiatry. In general medicine as well, informed consent had not yet developed into the modern doctrine we know today. In psychiatry, however, the gap was greater because refusal could be interpreted as a symptom and the patient might be hospitalized against his or her will.

As bioethics and patients' rights strengthened after the Second World War, particularly in response to abusive medical experimentation, the basic assumption changed. Treatment is not justified solely because a professional believes it will be beneficial. The person receiving care must, as far as possible, be a participant. In mental health, this change still confronts a difficult exception: what happens when the ability to consent is impaired?

The twentieth century added something to psychiatry that had not previously existed with the same intensity: therapeutic optimism. When new tools appear, there is a strong desire to use them. A physician who encountered a person in severe psychosis before the era of medications sometimes faced extremely limited options; when a treatment appeared promising, the very possibility of changing the course of illness could be experienced as a breakthrough. From the perspective of the period, doing nothing could seem no less dangerous than acting.

Yet therapeutic optimism also changes the balance of power. The more convinced the system becomes that it possesses a beneficial treatment, the more easily patient resistance can be perceived as an obstacle to overcome. If treatment is considered necessary, refusal may be seen as a result of illness rather than as a decision that has meaning in its own right. Here arises a tension that remains present in modern medicine: how to distinguish a situation in which illness genuinely impairs decision-making from a situation in which a person understands the information but evaluates the costs and benefits differently.

Historical judgment requires caution. It is easy to examine old treatments through today's knowledge and see only their risks, while professionals often acted in the face of enormous suffering and uncertainty. Recognizing this does not absolve systems of responsibility; it teaches a different lesson. Contemporary medicine also acts on incomplete knowledge, and treatments regarded today as advanced may be viewed differently decades from now. Rights such as informed consent, review, documentation, and freedom to refuse are therefore not obstacles to medical progress. They are mechanisms that protect people against excessive professional confidence - even when that confidence arises from good intentions.

The new professionalism also changed the figure of the psychiatrist. From a physician whose main role was to manage an institution and supervise daily order, the psychiatrist gradually became a specialist expected to diagnose, measure, choose treatment, and follow outcomes. This was an important step toward a more evidence-oriented medicine, but it also created a new distance between professional knowledge and the person's knowledge of himself or herself. History shows that both kinds of knowledge are necessary: the physician may know what research says about the probability of response; the person knows what price he or she is willing to pay to obtain it. Only when those forms of knowledge meet can treatment truly become shared.

The most important change, therefore, is not a simple transition from 'bad treatments' to 'good treatments.' It is a transition from a model in which the existence of an effective intervention itself provided broad justification for using it, to a model in which efficacy is only one question. Alongside it stand questions of risk, alternatives, personal values, capacity, and consent. This is the movement from medicine that seeks to do something to the patient toward medicine that must explain why, when, and under what conditions it is legitimate to do so.

The technologies of the twentieth century changed not only what psychiatry could do, but also what society expected from it. An institution that had once been primarily a place of supervision and custody gradually became a hospital expected to demonstrate outcomes: reduce symptoms, shorten hospitalization, and enable return to community life. Such a change creates new responsibilities. When treatment exists, failing to provide it may be regarded as neglect; but when treatment has significant adverse effects, providing it without discussing the cost becomes more problematic as well.

The gap between professional hope and personal experience is especially visible when treatment succeeds by one measure and fails by another. A physician may observe a reduction in delusional thinking and define that as improvement, while the patient reports fatigue, emotional blunting, or loss of ability to work. The two descriptions do not necessarily contradict each other. They measure different things. Modern medicine gradually learned that it is not enough to ask whether a symptom has diminished; one must also ask what has happened to the life in which that symptom existed.

This is also why the history of treatments that were abandoned or substantially modified matters. It should not be used to cast suspicion on every innovation, but to remind us that a medical system can be wrong even when it is confident in its intentions. Mechanisms of consent, follow-up, and documentation are not expressions of distrust in physicians. They are the means through which a profession learns to live with the possibility that its knowledge is incomplete. The more powerful the therapeutic tool, the more important that recognition becomes.

This question will accompany the rest of the book. Before turning to models of partnership, however, we must understand how law itself for many years provided a legitimate framework for deprivation of liberty. Medicine offered the diagnosis; the state gave it power. The next chapter examines the legal justifications for that power and the beginnings of constitutional critique.

Chapter Five

The Law Legitimizes the Deprivation of Liberty

Medicine Is Not Enough to Confine

Even if a physician is convinced that a person needs hospitalization, deprivation of liberty is an exercise of governmental power. It changes the person's legal position: the person is not free to go home, choose another setting, or end the intervention. Every modern legal system therefore requires a lawful source of authority.

This requirement was not always self-evident. In earlier periods, confinement in an institution could rest largely on a decision by a family, physician, or local authority. As the idea of the rule of law developed, it became clearer that even an action undertaken in the name of treatment had to be limited by law. Dedicated mental-health statutes therefore emerged, defining who could order hospitalization, under what circumstances, and for how long.

The existence of a law, however, does not itself guarantee rights. Law can regulate and limit power, but it can also grant broad legitimacy to that power. The important questions are therefore what conditions the law requires and what mechanisms of review it provides.

One of the classical legal justifications for intervention is patriae parens - the role of the state in protecting a person who is unable to care for himself or herself. The historical origin of the concept was not specifically psychiatric, but it fit easily with situations in which a person was regarded as incapable of making decisions.

Morally, this justification has considerable force. A society cannot ignore an unconscious person, a child, or someone who is unable to understand an immediate danger. In mental health as well, there are circumstances in which intervention expresses responsibility rather than oppression. The difficulty lies in the boundary of expansion. If psychiatric diagnosis itself is treated as proof of incapacity, protection becomes a mechanism for replacing a person's wishes across the board.

Modern rights-based law therefore tries to break the question down. Instead of asking, 'Is the person mentally ill?', it asks: Is there a concrete impairment in the ability to make this particular decision? Is the risk serious? Is there a way to support decision-making rather than replace it? And is the intervention as short and limited as possible?

Another justification is the state's authority to protect the public. If a person poses a serious and concrete danger to others, the state has authority to act. Yet here too a problem of equality arises. A person without a psychiatric diagnosis is not detained merely because of a vague concern that he or she might be dangerous in the future. Why should a mental-health diagnosis open a broader preventive pathway?

The traditional answer is that certain mental disorders can affect judgment and behavioral control, and that dangerousness related to such impairment justifies a distinct mechanism. Critics argue that creating a special legal regime on the basis of psychosocial or mental disability imposes burdens for which there is no full equivalent in the general population.

This debate became especially important after the Convention on the Rights of Persons with Disabilities. If equality means that disability itself cannot justify deprivation of liberty, legal models in which diagnosis is a necessary element of the grounds for detention must be reconsidered. Many health systems, however, argue that removing the specialized framework without building an alternative could impair the ability to protect people in severe crises.

One important development during the twentieth century was a gradual move away from models based largely on the existence of mental illness toward models that also require dangerousness, serious treatment need, or substantial impairment of judgment. The purpose was to limit the ability to hospitalize a person merely because his or her way of life was unconventional or because the system believed treatment would be beneficial.

The United States produced several of the most influential judicial decisions. In O'Connor v. Donaldson, the case concerned Kenneth Donaldson, who had been held for almost fifteen years in a state hospital in Florida. In 1975, the Supreme Court held that a state could not continue to confine a person who was not dangerous and who could live safely in freedom, alone or with the help of responsible family members or friends, merely because of mental illness. The decision did not abolish involuntary hospitalization, but it set a constitutional limit: diagnosis alone is not enough.

In Addington v. Texas in 1979, the Supreme Court held that civil involuntary commitment involves such a significant deprivation of liberty and carries such serious stigma that an ordinary preponderance-of-the-evidence standard is insufficient. A standard of 'clear and convincing evidence' is required. Here too the message was twofold: the state has authority to intervene, but because of the gravity of the intervention it must satisfy heightened evidentiary and procedural requirements.

Europe: Liberty Under Article 5

In the same year, 1979, the European Court of Human Rights delivered its judgment in Winterwerp v. the Netherlands. The decision became a cornerstone of European law on psychiatric detention. The Court articulated three central elements: the existence of a genuine mental disorder must be reliably established on the basis of objective medical expertise; the disorder must be of a kind or degree that warrants compulsory confinement; and continued confinement is justified only for as long as the relevant disorder persists.

The importance of Winterwerp lies not only in these conditions. It explicitly brought psychiatry into the language of human rights. Hospitalization was no longer a professional decision assessed solely by a medical standard; it was a deprivation of liberty examined under the European Convention on Human Rights. From this follows a right to effective legal review of continued detention.

Legal representation, a review committee, or a court may appear to be procedural matters unrelated to treatment. In practice, they alter the balance of power. A person who may review material, be heard, present evidence or an expert opinion, receive representation, and appeal is not entirely dependent on the institution that holds him or her.

Procedures do not prevent every error. Review bodies can become routine, representation can become formalistic, and judicial review may give substantial deference to professional assessment. Yet the very possibility that someone outside the institution will ask 'Why?' is one of the principal differences between a paternalistic institution and a system that seeks to respect rights.

Later in the book we will see how Israel's 1991 law created psychiatric review committees and appeal mechanisms, and how legal representation in involuntary hospitalization was expanded in the 2000s. This development illustrates that protection of rights is not a one-time event achieved by enacting a single statute. It is built in layers of authority, procedure, review, and resources.

At the same time, the opposite mistake must be avoided. A court cannot replace a psychiatrist, and legal procedure cannot provide treatment. A legal decision may determine that continued hospitalization is unlawful, but it does not create housing, home-based treatment, or support for the family. If the person is released into a situation in which no services exist, the right to liberty can become empty in practice.

Here the relationship between negative and positive rights becomes visible again. The right not to be unlawfully confined is a negative right - a limit on state power. The right to receive services that make community living possible is a positive right - a demand that the state act and invest. A genuine rights revolution needs both.

From Legitimization to Critique

The law's difficulty begins with the fact that it must make a binary decision in a world of probabilities. A court or quasi-judicial body must ultimately decide whether a person will remain hospitalized or be released, while professionals themselves can generally speak only in terms of higher or lower risk. No judge knows how the scenario that was not chosen would have unfolded. If a person is released and nothing happens, one cannot know whether the release was objectively safe or whether the risk simply did not materialize. If tragedy occurs, hindsight makes it easy to treat the outcome as proof that it was predictable.

The human tendency to infer the quality of a decision from its outcome creates structural pressure toward over-caution. From the system's perspective, an unnecessary hospitalization rarely receives the same public attention as a discharge followed by harm. For the individual, however, an 'error on the side of caution' is still an error with a price: days or weeks of lost liberty, disruption of work and family life, and damage to trust. The law must therefore protect against a risk that does not make headlines - the risk that the state will restrict too many people because it cannot be certain which of them will actually come to harm.

This is where procedure matters. The right to be heard, to receive representation, to know what is alleged, to examine relevant material, and to subject a decision to review does not guarantee that every decision will be correct. It does something different: it requires the system to slow down, give reasons, and expose itself to the possibility that it may be wrong. Sometimes the presence of an additional person who is not part of the treatment team changes the conversation. That person can ask whether an alternative exists, whether the behavior relied upon is still current, and whether the reason for continued hospitalization is truly risk or mainly difficulty finding an appropriate community placement.

Legal procedure also influences the experience of justice. People are more likely to accept difficult decisions when they feel they were given a genuine opportunity to speak and when reasons were explained to them. In this sense, procedural fairness is not only a constitutional principle but can also have therapeutic significance. It does not transform coercion into consent, but it can prevent coercion from being experienced as arbitrary and faceless.

Law enters psychiatry because liberty has a cost that is not only medical. A person hospitalized involuntarily may lose workdays, miss caring for children, become exposed before neighbors or colleagues, and carry afterward the knowledge that the state prevented him or her from leaving a particular place. These harms do not appear in a clinical symptom scale. The legal question therefore cannot disappear within medical assessment, even where that assessment is professional and well reasoned.

One of the deepest difficulties is the asymmetry between errors. When a person is released and tragedy occurs, the decision is immediately scrutinized: who knew, who warned, why was it not prevented? When a person is hospitalized unnecessarily and nothing dramatic occurs, there is rarely a comparable event forcing the system to reexamine itself. Liberty deprived 'just to be safe' leaves no clear headline. Precisely for this reason, law must also give weight to the quiet harm of excessive caution.

Fair procedure is intended to address that asymmetry. It brings into the process someone whose role is to ask questions that may be uncomfortable for the treating system: What is the factual basis? What has changed? Is there an alternative? Is there information that contradicts the assessment? The aim is not to turn every clinical decision into a legal confrontation. It is to ensure that when a clinical decision becomes a deprivation of liberty, it can also withstand the language of reasons, evidence, and review. In this sense, law does not stand outside treatment; it defines the conditions under which involuntary treatment and detention can be legitimate in a democratic society.

For much of the twentieth century, law provided a legal framework for the institutional psychiatric model. Gradually, particularly from the 1960s and 1970s onward, it also began to place limits on that model. This change occurred alongside social, research-based, and political criticism of the institutions themselves. To understand why the public and the law began asking harder questions, we must enter the human cost of life in the closed institution.

Chapter Six

The Human Cost of the Closed Institution

When Hospitalization Becomes a Way of Life

A brief hospitalization during a crisis can be protective. A person may receive a safe environment, intensive treatment, observation, and respite from overwhelming external pressures. Historically, however, a psychiatric institution was not always a place of days or weeks. For many people it became a place of months, years, and sometimes decades.

When hospitalization becomes a way of life, its effects are not merely medical. A person loses a previous routine, employment, relationships, property, privacy, and social roles. Children may grow up without a parent; partnerships may break apart; everyday skills may erode. Even if the original reason for hospitalization was severe illness, the cumulative consequences of institutional life create a new problem: how can a person return to a life that was never allowed to continue?

Sociological and psychiatric research described the phenomenon of institutionalization - not simply being present in an institution, but behavioral and social change resulting from adaptation to a life in which others make decisions. A person is not required to choose when to get up, what to cook, where to go, or how to manage a budget. Abilities that are not used can weaken.

This dependence can become an interpretive trap. The patient struggles to manage independent life, and the institution concludes that continued hospitalization is necessary; yet part of the difficulty was created because the institution itself prevented opportunities to practice independence. This is where rehabilitation becomes crucial: to assess capacity for community living, people need genuine opportunities to exercise it, rather than being assessed only within an environment that neutralizes autonomy.

In a large institution, a person may become a chart, a bed, or a diagnosis. This is not necessarily the result of malice. Overburdened systems need classification, procedures, and documentation. Yet when the system sees the diagnosis before the person, individual choices become secondary.

Privacy is a clear example. Shared rooms, examinations, observation, restrictions on belongings, monitoring of movement, and broad access to medical information can shrink a person's personal boundaries. Some restrictions are necessary for safety; others arise from institutional convenience. Distinguishing between them is one of the tasks of a rights-based system.

Dignity is not a luxury added to good treatment. It is part of treatment itself. A person who feels humiliated, powerless, or unheard may lose trust in staff and withdraw from cooperation. Reducing coercion can therefore be not only a moral objective but also a clinical one.

The psychiatric institution was not only a building. It was also a social marker. Hospitalization itself could attach an identity of 'madness' or 'dangerousness' to a person even after discharge. Stigma affects employment, housing, social relationships, intimate partnerships, and the willingness to seek help in the future.

The problem becomes more complex because stigma can be internalized. A person who repeatedly hears that he or she is incapable, cannot be trusted, or is defined by illness may absorb that message. The recovery model that would later develop seeks precisely to break this connection: diagnosis is not destiny, and recovery does not necessarily require the complete disappearance of every symptom in order for a person to live a meaningful life.

The term 'institutional violence' does not refer only to physical assault or intentional abuse. It can describe a system in which the structure itself produces harm: overcrowding, understaffing, routine use of restrictive measures, lack of access to personal belongings, long periods of inactivity, or decisions made without participation.

There is an important difference between an isolated incident and a pattern. A team may use restraint in a particular event because it feels there is no alternative. But if a particular ward uses restraint at a consistently high rate, the question is not only whether each individual event met the rules; it is whether the organization itself creates conditions that increase the need for coercion. Is staffing adequate? Are staff trained in de-escalation? Is the environment noisy or threatening? Is there a voluntary quiet space? Do patients know what to expect?

The shift from thinking about a 'violent patient' to thinking about an 'escalating encounter' is part of the modern change. It does not deny personal responsibility or genuine danger; it adds institutional responsibility.

Families have always occupied a complex role. At times they were the main force bringing a person to treatment and saving a life. At times they were also partners in hospitalization decisions in which insufficient weight was given to the person's wishes. Institutions sometimes treated the family as a source of information but not necessarily as an equal partner; in other cases, the family itself asked that the person remain institutionalized because it had no capacity to manage the situation at home.

A modern rights-based system cannot choose a simple side between the patient and the family. It must protect confidentiality and autonomy while also recognizing that family may be a central source of support. The challenge is to create agreements, boundaries, and tailored information-sharing rather than a system in which the family either knows everything or knows nothing.

One of the most important revolutions was not legal but epistemic: recognition that people who have experienced hospitalization and treatment possess knowledge that is no less important than professional knowledge, even if it is of a different kind. Movements of service users, psychiatric survivors, and people with lived experience demanded that others not speak about them without them.

Their accounts revealed gaps between therapeutic intention and lived experience. An intervention viewed by staff as 'calming' may be experienced as coercion. A hospitalization formally described as 'voluntary' may be experienced as having no real alternative. The tension does not prove that one side is wrong; it teaches that treatment is measured not only by what professionals intended to do, but also by what the person experienced.

End of an Era or a Change of Form?

From the 1950s onward, many countries began reducing large psychiatric institutions. New medications, economic costs, public criticism, judicial decisions, and civil-rights movements all contributed to deinstitutionalization. Yet the institution did not disappear entirely, and institutional power can also exist in the community when services are built primarily around monitoring, conditions, and compliance.

The next transition in this book is therefore not simply 'from institution to freedom.' It is a move from criticism of the institution toward attempts to build another model - community-based treatment, rights, due process, and rehabilitation. Some efforts succeeded; others created new problems. The next chapter examines the movements that challenged the basic assumptions of institutional psychiatry and sought to shift the center of gravity from the expert to the person.

The deepest cost of prolonged institutional life is not always the dramatic event that is easiest to describe. Sometimes it accumulates precisely through the small things that disappear. The ability to choose what to wear, when to make coffee, whom to speak with, whether to go for a walk, or how to arrange a room may seem trivial compared with questions of diagnosis and treatment. Yet human life is built largely from choices of exactly this kind. When they are taken away over time, the person does not lose only legal liberty; he or she may lose the sense of being the author of his or her own life.

Time itself also takes on a different character in an institution. Outside, a week is measured by meetings, work, errands, family events, and plans. Inside, it may be measured by meals, medication rounds, physician visits, and scheduled access to the courtyard. For someone who spends months or years in such a setting, this rhythm can make discharge itself frightening. Life outside the ward requires decisions, initiative, and coping with uncertainty - precisely the things the institution has spared or prevented. From this emerges the paradox of 'institutional dependence': the system seeks to prepare a person for independent life, while the conditions within it may weaken the skills independence requires.

The family undergoes a parallel process. At the beginning, hospitalization may feel like rescue: an end to sleepless nights, uncertainty, and fear. As hospitalization continues, the family may shift from being central to the person's daily life to becoming visitors during fixed hours. Sometimes this allows the family to recover; sometimes it weakens the relationship and the family's ability to participate in later rehabilitation. Criticism of the institution therefore cannot ignore the burden that led families to seek it in the first place. A society that reduces hospitalization without offering support to families simply transfers a heavy responsibility back to them.

The human cost of a closed institution is not measured only by the number of locked doors. It also reaches identity. People build identity through roles: parent, worker, neighbor, student, friend. Prolonged hospitalization narrows those roles and expands one role - 'patient.' The more the system organizes life around diagnosis, the easier it becomes for everything else to disappear from view. A person who was a carpenter, teacher, or musician before hospitalization may be understood within the institution mainly through behavior on the ward.

This narrowing also affects staff. A busy institution often rewards short, efficient information: who took medication, who slept, who went on leave, who became agitated. The things that make up a whole life - relationships, taste, history, fears, aspirations - can be pushed aside because they are harder to measure. This is not an accusation against individual professionals. It is an organizational tendency that appears in every large system, and it is why mechanisms are needed to return the person to his or her own story.

Accounts by former patients were important for exactly this reason. They added to the history of psychiatry information that medical records can barely capture: what a door sounds like when it closes from the outside, what it means to ask permission to use a telephone, and what it feels like when people speak about you in the third person while you are present. Such details are not 'too emotional' for legal discussion. They explain why rights such as privacy, information, and contact with the outside world are not decorative additions but protections against the disappearance of the person inside an institutional role.

Leaving the institution therefore requires more than opening a gate. A person needs a place to live, income, connection to health services, opportunities to work or study, relationships with people who are not professionals, and a sense of being wanted in public space. Without these, discharge may amount to formal freedom only. Recognition of this fact would later become one of the foundations of community rehabilitation.

Part Three

The Beginning of Change: From Institutions to Rights

Chapter Seven

The Critique of Psychiatry

When the Institution Became an Object of Criticism

By the middle of the twentieth century, psychiatry had already become an established medical profession, and psychiatric hospitals were a familiar component of the welfare state. It was precisely then that criticism widened. It came from different sources and did not rest on a single claim. Lawyers asked whether liberty could be taken away without due process; sociologists examined how institutions reshape the identities of those who live in them; psychiatrists themselves warned against paternalism; and people who had experienced hospitalization began to organize and describe the system from a perspective that had previously received little public attention.

Criticism was not the same as opposition to medicine. Some critics sought to improve psychiatry rather than abolish it. Others challenged the very idea that a medical institution should be able to define social deviance as illness. The term 'anti-psychiatry,' which became established in the discourse of the 1960s and 1970s, later grouped together highly diverse and sometimes opposing approaches. R. D. Laing, David Cooper, Thomas Szasz, and others did not share a single doctrine, and not all accepted the label. Yet they helped unsettle the assumption that the psychiatric system was merely a neutral mechanism of diagnosis and treatment.

One of the strongest questions raised by the critique was who has the authority to define normality. Every field of medicine needs definitions of disease, but in mental health the boundary between symptom, suffering, difference, and socially disapproved behavior can be especially complex. When a diagnosis carries with it the possibility of involuntary hospitalization, the question is not only scientific; it is also a question of power.

Historically, there are examples in which social norms influenced psychiatric categories. This does not prove that every diagnosis is a 'social invention,' as some radical critics argued. Severe mental disorders involve real suffering, functional impairment, and genuine clinical phenomena. The critique did, however, contribute to the understanding that diagnosis always exists within a culture, institutions, and language, and that the uses made of diagnosis beyond the clinical need must be examined carefully.

From a rights perspective, the implication is clear: a medical diagnosis cannot erase a person's legal personality. It should not automatically become a presumption that the person is dangerous, incapable, or unreliable. If a particular right must be restricted, that restriction should rest on an individualized and relevant assessment rather than on a global label.

Erving Goffman's study of total institutions profoundly influenced the way psychiatric hospitals were understood. Goffman did not focus on whether a particular diagnosis was correct, but on what the institution does to a person's identity. Life in a framework in which sleep, work, treatment, and leisure are all managed under one authority can create a new 'moral career': the person learns to see himself or herself through the categories offered by the institution.

The contribution of sociological criticism was to widen the field of vision. Treatment is not only the active ingredient in a medication or the content of a conversation. The environment is also an intervention. A locked door, institutional clothing, the manner in which a patient is addressed, access to a telephone, privacy, and the way decisions are made all influence a person's experience and rehabilitation.

This idea would reappear decades later in trauma-informed approaches and in efforts to reduce coercion. If a treatment environment can intensify fear, shame, or helplessness, it can also be designed to reduce them.

Thomas Szasz and the Debate over 'Mental Illness'

Thomas Szasz was among the most forceful critics of coercive psychiatry. He argued, among other things, that the concept of 'mental illness' could conceal moral and social judgments in medical language, and he opposed involuntary hospitalization in principle. His positions drew substantial criticism, particularly because they were seen as minimizing the medical and biological dimensions of severe disorders.

His importance to the rights debate does not depend on accepting all of his claims. He forced legal discourse to confront a basic question: can treatment that a person does not want still be called treatment in the same sense? And what is the difference between a physician who offers help and an institution that holds a person against his or her will?

Modern psychiatry need not choose between two extremes - 'every disorder is a simple biological disease' and 'mental illness does not exist.' Contemporary models recognize biological, psychological, and social components, as well as substantial heterogeneity among individuals. Yet the debate Szasz provoked remains relevant whenever diagnosis becomes the basis for exercising authority.

R. D. Laing sought to listen to the psychotic experience rather than merely classify it. He emphasized the meaning of relationships, family, and social context. Here too, parts of his thinking were criticized and psychiatric research moved in other directions. Yet culturally, the idea that behavior that appears meaningless from the outside may become understandable within the person's own world was important.

From this follows an insight that is both therapeutic and rights-based: before imposing an intervention, one should try to understand what the person is saying. Refusal of medication may stem from a delusional belief, but it may also stem from severe side effects experienced in the past. Fear of hospitalization may be part of paranoia, but it may also be a response to a traumatic hospitalization. If every objection is immediately translated into a symptom, the system loses essential information.

The deepest change occurred when people who had been patients began to speak for themselves. Movements of former patients, psychiatric survivors, and service users challenged a system in which physicians, researchers, and families spoke about the patient while the patient's own voice was barely heard.

They raised issues that professional literature had not always measured: humiliation, fear, loss of control, subtle pressure, sexual abuse in institutions, adverse effects, difficulty leaving the system, and the stigma attached to diagnosis itself. Alongside criticism, peer-support models also emerged - people with lived experience helping others through knowledge acquired from experience rather than professional training alone.

The phrase 'Nothing About Us Without Us' became a principle of the disability-rights movement, but in mental health it has a particular force. If a person may lose liberty in the name of treatment, there is an increased obligation to include people who have experienced the system in designing its rules.

A Critique That Does Not Abolish Treatment

A balanced discussion requires a distinction between criticism of power and denial of suffering. People with severe mental disorders may require intensive treatment and may sometimes themselves seek the protection of hospitalization. Families can face extremely difficult situations in which community services are insufficient. Staff members often work under conditions of risk and scarcity.

Historical criticism does not mean that the solution is to leave a person alone in the name of liberty. It means that treatment must also be examined from the perspective of the person receiving it, that coercion requires a weighty justification, and that a system is measured in part by its ability to build alternatives before a crisis reaches its peak.

The power of the critique also came from changing the identity of those authorized to speak about psychiatry. For many years, knowledge was defined almost entirely from above: a physician described symptoms, an institution documented behavior, and lawyers examined authority. When people who had experienced hospitalization began to articulate their own experience, another form of knowledge appeared - not instead of clinical knowledge, but alongside it. Questions such as fear, humiliation, loss of control, and mistrust became part of professional discussion rather than merely personal complaints.

This development challenged a deep assumption: that once a person is diagnosed as ill, what he or she says can be viewed primarily through the diagnosis. A person who resists hospitalization may be characterized as having 'no insight'; a person who says that treatment caused harm may be treated as someone who does not understand the medical necessity. Service-user and psychiatric-survivor movements sought to reverse this direction of interpretation. Even if intervention was justified, they argued, the person's experience does not disappear. It is possible to say at the same time that the staff tried to save a life and that the way the intervention was carried out left trauma.

Criticism itself, however, can also become simplistic. Not every hospitalization is oppression, not every medication is an instrument of control, and not every mental condition can be resolved through social acceptance alone. Many people report that medication, hospitalization, or a protected setting enabled them to return to life. Taking rights seriously does not require denial of illness or severe suffering. It requires holding two things together: recognizing the need for treatment while asking how therapeutic power is exercised and by whom.

This change slowly entered training and research as well. The patient's experience, once appearing mainly as a clinical description of symptoms, began to be studied as a question in its own right: how hospitalization is experienced, what makes a person feel heard, and what helps a person return to functioning. This does not replace medical outcomes; it broadens the question of what counts as a good outcome. If treatment reduces symptoms but leaves a person convinced that he or she will never seek help again, it is difficult to call the result a complete success.

A significant change in professional language followed. Instead of a binary argument between 'psychiatry' and 'anti-psychiatry,' discourse developed around partnership, choice, recovery, trauma, and rights. This language is less dramatic than a call to close every institution, but institutionally it is more radical: it seeks to change the power relations within treatment itself.

The critique of psychiatry was not one movement and did not speak with one voice. Some critics sought to abolish large institutions while retaining confidence in psychiatric medicine. Others challenged the authority to define an experience as 'illness' in the first place. Some focused mainly on civil rights, others on power relations, and still others on participation in treatment decisions. Blending these voices sometimes produced a caricature in which all criticism was labeled 'anti-psychiatry,' even though the internal disagreements were profound.

The differences among the critics teach an important lesson. A system need not accept every claim in order to learn from criticism. One can reject the claim that mental disorder does not exist while agreeing that diagnosis can become a label. One can recognize the effectiveness of medication while still requiring consent and choice. One can accept the need for hospitalization in some situations while listening seriously to accounts of harm during hospitalization. The ability to hold these tensions is a mark of professional maturity.

Over time, knowledge based on lived experience also changed status. Former patients no longer accepted merely having their 'story heard' at a symbolic event; they sought participation in service planning, staff training, and research. The move from testimony to partnership changes the question of who counts as an expert. It does not replace professional training, but adds knowledge that cannot be acquired from a textbook. A person who has experienced coercion knows something about coercion that a professional can learn only by being willing to listen.

The first practical transition that attempted to apply this critique on a large scale was deinstitutionalization. It sought to move the center of gravity from the hospital to the community. As the next chapter shows, however, opening the gates of the institution was only the beginning of the task.

Chapter Eight

The Deinstitutionalization Revolution

Not a Single Event but a Global Process

'Deinstitutionalization' can sound like a simple act: close institutions and release people into the community. In practice, it was a prolonged process that differed from country to country and involved several movements at once: reducing beds in large institutions, shortening hospital stays, developing outpatient treatment, housing and rehabilitation, and shifting resources from inpatient systems to community systems.

The causes were many. Antipsychotic medications made treatment outside the institution more realistic for many people. The cost of maintaining large institutions weighed heavily on states. Public and legal criticism strengthened demands for liberty. An ideology of normalization and rights sought to enable people to live in the community rather than in a parallel world reserved for the 'mentally ill.'

The pace at which beds were closed, however, did not always match the pace at which services were built. That gap largely determined whether deinstitutionalization became a process of liberation or abandonment.

The introduction of chlorpromazine and other medications in the 1950s contributed to the ability to reduce acute symptoms and make discharge possible. Medication, however, does not replace housing, employment, relationships, psychological treatment, or daily support. A person may be clinically stable yet still be unable to rent an apartment, find work, or manage life after years in an institution.

When systems treated medication as the solution to deinstitutionalization, they underestimated the scale of social need. In some countries the result was a 'revolving door': brief hospitalization, discharge without adequate support, another crisis, and another hospitalization. In other cases people moved from psychiatric institutions to other institutional settings - nursing homes, welfare facilities, or the prison system. This process is sometimes called transinstitutionalization: the institution changes form rather than disappearing.

In the United States, deinstitutionalization is a particularly complex example. The development of medications, judicial decisions limiting commitment, federal policy, and changes in financing all contributed to a dramatic reduction in state-hospital beds. Community mental health centers were developed at the same time. Yet the community system did not always receive resources sufficient to meet the need. Historical research indicates that the failure to build a strong community system contributed to people with severe mental disorders becoming homeless or repeatedly entering the criminal justice system. The retrospective question should therefore not be simply 'Was deinstitutionalization a mistake?' but 'What kind of deinstitutionalization was carried out?' Reducing institutions without services is not equivalent to a planned transition to community care.

Italy became a symbol of radical reform. The work of Franco Basaglia and the Psichiatria Democratica movement challenged the psychiatric institution itself as a structure that produces exclusion. In 1978, Law 180, identified with Basaglia, halted new admissions to traditional psychiatric hospitals and promoted community services and small psychiatric units in general hospitals.

The Italian experience was not uniform. Trieste became an international example of a comparatively open community system, while other regions struggled to develop services. Studies over the years have identified both major achievements and significant gaps. Italy's importance lies in the fact that the reform was framed not only as a matter of efficiency but as a matter of citizenship: the person does not 'belong' to a psychiatric institution; the person is a citizen whom the community must enable to live within it.

This principle would recur in rehabilitation legislation in Israel and in the Convention on the Rights of Persons with

Disabilities: living in the community is not an act of charity but a component of equality and participation.

In other countries the process was more gradual. Large hospitals were reduced, community services were built, and psychiatric hospitalization was partly transferred to general hospitals. Community treatment teams, housing frameworks, and day services developed alongside these changes.

The differences among models show that there is no single formula. A country with a strong welfare network, public housing, and accessible community services can reduce hospitalization differently from a country in which the family is almost the only source of support. Culture, financing, the structure of the healthcare system, and law all shape whether the community can become a genuine alternative.

Deinstitutionalization illustrates the distinction between two meanings of liberty. Negative liberty is freedom from coercion: not being held behind a locked door. Positive liberty is the practical ability to live, choose, and participate. A person discharged from a hospital but left without housing, treatment, or income is not confined, yet the range of real choices remains severely restricted.

A central principle follows: reducing coercion requires investment. It is relatively easy to write in law that hospitalization is a last resort. It is far harder to fund home treatment, crisis teams, supported housing, and services available twenty-four hours a day. If alternatives do not exist, the 'last resort' can in practice become the only resort.

Community-based services can also be coercive. A compulsory outpatient treatment order, conditions attached to housing, close monitoring, or pressure to take medication can transfer power from the ward to the home. Some argue that community coercion prevents hospitalization and permits greater liberty; others regard it as an extension of coercive psychiatry into ordinary life.

The judgment depends on the details: the threshold for an order, its duration, rights of appeal, what happens if the person refuses, and whether the order is accompanied by services the person actually sought. Coercion without services is mainly surveillance; services without choice can become paternalism. The ideal model seeks to make support so accessible and dependable that the need for coercion diminishes.

The Lesson of Deinstitutionalization

The lesson is neither to return to large institutions nor to assume that every hospitalization is a failure. It is to understand that a mental-health system is a continuum. A person should be able to receive early help in the community, intensive treatment during crisis, hospitalization when necessary, and rehabilitation afterward - without falling between systems.

When the continuum is missing, hospitals become blocked by people who have nowhere to be discharged, emergency departments become the gateway to care, and families carry burdens they cannot bear alone. When the continuum exists, hospitalization can become a short and focused intervention rather than a way of life.

Deinstitutionalization exposed an uncomfortable truth: it is easier to close a bed than to build a community. A bed is a clear organizational unit, with a budget, staff, and a physical place. Life in the community depends on an entire network - housing, employment, primary care, psychiatry, welfare services, transportation, income, and social support. If one link is missing, a person may move between emergency rooms, temporary settings, and family homes that cannot carry the burden alone.

Where institutions were reduced before alternatives were built, some people did not truly move from an institution into liberty but from one institution to other institutions: shelters, rigid residential frameworks, prisons, or life on the street. This shows that not every place physically located 'in the community' is community-based in spirit. An apartment in which every decision is dictated by staff can reproduce institutional patterns even without a gate or guard. By contrast, a setting with intensive support can promote independence if it is built around choice, privacy, and personal goals.

The move into the community also changed the role of the clinician. In a hospital it is comparatively easy to know who is responsible: the team is on site and the patient is accessible. In the community, responsibility is dispersed. A person may see a physician every few weeks, a rehabilitation worker elsewhere, and a social worker in another framework. The advantage is that life is not conducted inside one institution; the disadvantage is the risk that no one sees the whole picture. This is why continuity of care, coordination, and crisis services capable of reaching the person - rather than merely waiting for the person to arrive - are so important.

For families, the change was sometimes a quiet revolution. A relative who in the past would have remained for years in an institution returned home, and much of the responsibility moved into the family living room. Where good services were built, the return enabled relationships and community life. Where services were lacking, the family effectively became a ward without staff. Family organizations therefore demanded something more than a choice between institution and abandonment: support that allows closeness without turning relatives into sole caregivers twenty-four hours a day.

Successful deinstitutionalization is therefore not measured by the number of beds closed. It is measured by what happened to people afterward: whether they live where they choose, whether they have meaningful relationships, whether they receive treatment in time, and whether crisis repeatedly sends them back to the same door that reform intended to move them beyond.

Deinstitutionalization succeeded where closure of institutions was accompanied by the construction of alternatives, and failed where discharge came before services. This distinction matters because public debate tends to measure success by the number of beds eliminated. Bed numbers are easy to count; the quality of life of those who left is far more complex. A person can be 'in the community' and still live in isolation, without continuous treatment and without a stable place. In such a situation, community is a geographical location rather than a framework of citizenship.

In several countries, a pattern appeared in which people moved from one institution to another: those who did not receive adequate mental-health and community services found themselves in homeless shelters, prisons, or general emergency departments. One need not accept the term 'transinstitutionalization' literally to understand the danger. If a system closes a psychiatric institution without building housing and support, it does not eliminate the need; it transfers it to another system, often one less suited to meeting it.

The lesson of deinstitutionalization is therefore neither nostalgia for the large institution nor longing for an era in which people were held for years behind a gate. The lesson is that liberty has an infrastructure. It requires a home, income, treatment, relationships, and services that can be obtained before a situation becomes an emergency. Where this infrastructure exists, reducing institutions can be liberation. Where it is absent, the same reform may feel to the person like abandonment in the name of rights.

The move from institution to community became linked in the 1970s, 1980s, and 1990s with a parallel development: the transformation of human rights into an explicit legal framework for mental health. That is the subject of the next chapter.

Chapter Nine

Human Rights Enter Psychiatry

From Benevolence to Right

There is a profound difference between a system that says, 'A patient should be treated with dignity,' and a system that says, 'A patient has a right to dignity.' In the first, dignity depends on professional ethics and culture; in the second, it becomes a legal standard that can be demanded of the state and the institution.

After the Second World War, international human-rights law developed rapidly. The Universal Declaration of Human Rights of 1948 and the international conventions that followed established a language of dignity, liberty, equality, privacy, and health. For a long time, people with disabilities - especially psychosocial disabilities - were not central to the formulation of these rules. Gradually, however, it became clear that universal rights also apply inside hospitals and institutions.

The implication was revolutionary: a person does not lose rights because of hospitalization, and a diagnosis does not create a zone in which law ceases to operate.

The right to liberty was the first to receive strong legal expression in relation to psychiatric hospitalization. Article 5 of the European Convention on Human Rights allows, under certain conditions, deprivation of liberty on grounds related to mental disorder, but the European Court of Human Rights turned that exception into a framework of scrutiny. Winterwerp and the case law that followed required a medical basis, continuing justification, and access to a procedure capable of reviewing the detention.

In the United States, requirements of due process developed in parallel. Procedures for involuntary commitment were increasingly required to recognize the gravity of the deprivation of liberty and the stigma attached to it. The change did not abolish state authority; it reversed the presumption. The state had to justify why a person was not free, rather than requiring the person to prove why release was deserved.

Rights do not end at the hospital gate. Even when hospitalization itself is lawful, questions remain about privacy, communication, visits, clothing, searches of personal belongings, access to medical information, respectful treatment, and protection from harm.

A safe system may need restrictions, but every restriction should be related to a purpose. A ban on telephone use, for example, should not be automatic if risk can be managed individually. A search should not become humiliation. Medical information should not be disclosed beyond what is necessary. When a person is dependent on an institution, even 'small rules' carry substantial weight.

The right to dignity requires attention to the manner of intervention, not only its goal. A necessary act can be performed respectfully or humiliatingly. A person can be told what is happening even when he or she disagrees. The person can be allowed to ask questions, contact a lawyer or a trusted person, and participate in the decision as far as possible.

In 1991, the United Nations General Assembly adopted the Principles for the Protection of Persons with Mental Illness and for the Improvement of Mental Health Care. The principles were an important step for their time. They addressed standards of care, consent, confidentiality, rights within institutions, and conditions for involuntary admission.

From the later perspective of the Convention on the Rights of Persons with Disabilities, however, the 1991 Principles are now regarded as limited because they still permit comparatively broad intervention based on mental disability. The difference between the two instruments illustrates the evolution of the discourse: from an effort to make coercion more humane and better supervised, toward the question of whether using disability itself as a basis for deprivation of rights is compatible with equality.

One possible error is to argue that because a person has a right to health, the state may compel treatment in order to realize that right. Rights do not operate in that way. The right to health requires availability, accessibility, quality, and appropriateness of services, but it does not cancel bodily integrity or consent.

The tension is real when a person refuses life-saving treatment because a disorder impairs judgment. Yet any resolution of that tension must be specific and proportionate. It cannot turn the right to health into a general justification for replacing a person's will.

On the contrary, a rights-based system should ask whether the person could have received voluntary treatment earlier. Long waiting times, cost, stigma, and services that are not culturally appropriate can mean that the first encounter with the system occurs only after a crisis has become severe. In such a situation, coercion is not solely a result of illness; it may also be the result of failure of access.

The right to legal representation changes the status of a hospitalized person. A lawyer is not there to decide whether treatment is clinically good; the lawyer's role is to ensure that the law is followed, that the person understands the procedure, and that the person's voice is heard. Even when a review body concludes that hospitalization is justified, the presence of independent advocacy reduces the risk that the process becomes an automatic approval of the institution's position.

Different systems have developed models of legal assistance, independent advocates, or patient representatives. The differences reflect varying conceptions of the role: should the representative express the person's wishes even when the representative believes those wishes may cause harm, or may the representative act according to the person's 'best interests'? In a strong rights-based framework, the starting point is representation of the person's will and preferences rather than their replacement.

Equality: The Next Stage

The first stage of human rights in mental health focused mainly on protection from harm: do not hospitalize without legal conditions, do not use force without justification, and do not deny review. The next stage broadened the discussion to equality and participation.

A person with a psychosocial disability should not merely be protected from the institution; the person should have a real opportunity to work, study, live independently, form a family, and participate in the community. At this point mental health converges with the disability-rights movement.

The next major development at the international level would be the United Nations Convention on the Rights of Persons with Disabilities, which would later question the very link between psychosocial disability and deprivation of liberty. The Convention, the dates of its adoption, and its implications are examined in Chapter 27. Before that, the book turns to Israel itself: how the mental-health system was built, what legal world the 1955 law created, and why a new law was needed in 1991.

The move to a language of rights gradually changed the room in which decisions were made. In the past, the central question was what the physician thought should be done. In a rights-based framework, that medical question remains important, but additional questions enter the room: What does the person want? What does the person understand? What is the less restrictive alternative? Who represents the person? How can the decision be challenged? Each question introduces another voice and reduces the possibility that one conclusion will be treated as an unquestionable truth.

Rights also require infrastructure. A right to representation is not meaningful if no representative can arrive in time; a right of appeal loses force if the hearing takes place only after hospitalization has already ended; a right to information is not realized when the explanation is written in language the person cannot understand during crisis. This is what distinguishes rights law from a moral declaration. Rights must be translated into procedures, forms, timetables, training, and staffing.

This has special importance in psychiatry because the person whose rights are being protected may at that moment be confused, frightened, or suspicious. It is precisely then that it becomes easy to treat a right as a 'burden' interfering with treatment. Yet a right is tested not when respecting it is convenient but when doing so requires effort. A slow explanation to an agitated person, another attempt to hear the person's position, finding an interpreter, or waiting briefly before an irreversible decision are small acts that reveal the difference between a system that recognizes rights on paper and one that treats them as a way of working.

Human rights also changed the question of who must prove what. In a paternalistic world, a person seeking to leave an institution sometimes had to show that he or she was 'worthy' of freedom. In a rights-based world, the presumption is reversed: liberty is the rule, and the state must justify the exception. This may appear to be a legal shift, but it has a deep effect on professional language. Instead of asking why release would be advisable, one asks why continued detention is permissible.

The right to due process also acquired practical meaning. A person in crisis is not always able to activate rights independently. A long document explaining a right of appeal is of little use if it is handed over while the person is frightened and does not understand his or her status. Rights therefore must be translated into working conditions: a short explanation, repetition of information, an available representative, an interpreter, time for conversation, and a review body capable of convening while the decision still matters.

This reveals the difference between proclaiming rights and organizing rights. The first can stop at principles. The second requires schedules, budgets, and responsibility. Especially in mental health, where a person may be confused or suspicious, the system cannot place the entire burden of activating safeguards on the individual. In this sense, the right to liberty is not only the right to say 'no'; it is the right to a system capable of hearing that 'no' and examining it even when it is spoken in crisis.

The new discourse did not abolish paternalism overnight. It created a continuing competition between two languages. One speaks of responsibility, protection, and dangerousness; the other of liberty, choice, and dignity. Modern legislation tries to connect them, not always successfully. This tension stands at the center of the Israeli story.

Part Four

Israel: From the Early State to the Treatment of Mental Patients Law

Chapter Ten

Mental Health in Mandatory Palestine and the Early Years of the State

Before Statehood: Care, Charity, and Institutions

The history of mental health in the Land of Israel did not begin with the establishment of the state, nor is it a simple story of moving from an absence of care to a modern medical system. During the Ottoman period and the British Mandate, frameworks already existed for people experiencing severe mental distress. Some grew from community and philanthropic initiatives, while others were connected to governmental structures. As in Europe and North America, the boundary between treatment, supervision, and separation from society was often blurred.

By the end of the nineteenth century and the beginning of the twentieth, a more medical understanding of mental disorders began to take root. Alongside charitable institutions, services gradually developed around medical expertise and the distinction between physical and mental illness. During the Mandate, governmental mechanisms were added, including the government mental hospital in Bethlehem. This system did not develop in a vacuum: it reflected tensions among local traditions of care, Jewish and Arab institutions, European psychiatric knowledge, and colonial administration.

Already at this stage a pattern emerged that would accompany the mental-health system after statehood. A person in severe mental distress was viewed at the same time as someone needing treatment and as someone who might disrupt family or public order. The question of hospitalization was therefore never purely medical. It also involved the family, the community, the police, public authorities, and society's ability to tolerate unusual behavior outside an institution.

With the establishment of the State of Israel in 1948, the health system had to cope within a short period with enormous population growth, mass immigration, shortages of infrastructure, and shortages of trained professionals. Mental health was part of that challenge. The need was not only for more beds but also for professional services, workforce training, and legal regulation of situations in which a person did not agree to treatment or hospitalization.

In the state's early years, psychiatric hospitalization was a central component of care. This was consistent with the dominant international thinking of the period: the psychiatric hospital was seen as a place where treatment could be provided, people in severe conditions could be supervised, and, where necessary, a person perceived as dangerous to self or others could be separated from the community. Community treatment in the modern sense was far more limited.

The shortage of trained staff intensified dependence on institutions. When there are too few clinics, crisis teams, supported housing programs, home-treatment services, or rehabilitation services, the practical response to severe crisis becomes binary: the person remains at home, sometimes without adequate support, or enters a hospital. In such circumstances the hospital is not merely one treatment option; it becomes the center of gravity of the entire system.

Immigration, Trauma, and a Society Under Construction

A young society built after war, absorbing Holocaust survivors and immigrants from many countries while coping with poverty, overcrowding, and cultural gaps, also carried a considerable psychological burden. Yet recognition of mental distress was not always straightforward. A national ethos of building, work, military service, and recovery could encourage resilience, but it could also make psychological vulnerability difficult to speak about.

Stigma toward mental illness was substantial. Psychiatric hospitalization could be perceived not only as a medical event but as a social mark carried by the person and the family. Fear of labeling affected help-seeking, families' desire to conceal distress, and attitudes toward those discharged from institutions.

Historical judgment requires caution. Mental-health professionals in the 1950s worked under conditions very different from those of the twenty-first century. Knowledge, medications, welfare budgets, community services, and understandings of human rights were different. Historical understanding does not require approval of every practice accepted at the time. On the contrary, comparison between periods helps reveal the extent to which the definition of medical treatment is shaped by the values of its era.

By the middle of the 1950s, the need for dedicated Israeli legislation regulating psychiatric treatment and hospitalization had become clear. The problem was complex. On one hand, the state wanted to enable rapid intervention when a person required treatment but could not or would not consent. On the other hand, involuntary hospitalization is a deprivation of liberty, so the law needed to define who was authorized to order it and under what conditions.

When Health Minister Yosef Serlin presented the Mental Patients Treatment Bill to the Knesset in 1955, he described three dimensions of the problem: the scale of hospitalization, the shortage of psychiatric personnel, and the need to regulate the field by legislation. His remarks reflected a view characteristic of the period: a desire, as far as possible, to avoid a judicial process that might frighten the patient and the family, while at the same time preserving mechanisms intended to prevent abuse of hospitalization.

This formulation reveals the dilemma of the first law. The legislature sought to protect the person, but it did so within a system that gave substantial weight to medical authority and comparatively little weight to independent judicial review. From the perspective of 1955, this could appear humane and practical: fewer courts, less stigma, more treatment. From a contemporary human-rights perspective, however, the absence of strong independent process may itself create risk.

The family played a central role in the mental-health system of the period. When a person entered crisis, relatives were often the first to recognize the change and the first to manage its consequences. In the absence of a broad community system, the family carried a heavy burden: supervising, calming, seeking treatment, and sometimes agreeing to or requesting hospitalization.

This created a delicate tension among three centers of power: the individual, the family, and the state. At times their wishes coincided; at times they did not. A person might refuse hospitalization that the family regarded as essential. A family might request release while the clinical team believed the situation remained dangerous. The state had to decide when it would enter the family sphere and replace consent with coercion.

The 1955 law was born from this tension. To understand the transformation of 1991, the Patients' Rights Law, and modern discourse on autonomy, it is necessary to begin here: in a period in which the desire to protect and treat was often regarded as a sufficient reason to expand professional authority.

The Point of Transition

The early years of the state thus laid the foundations for an institutional psychiatric system and dedicated legislation. Yet those foundations rested on assumptions that today seem less self-evident: that the physician is the main authority who knows what is best for the patient; that hospitalization is the natural response to severe crisis; and that legal proceedings may interfere with treatment more than they protect rights.

The young Israeli system developed under conditions that made tailored services difficult to build. The state absorbed large populations, faced shortages of housing and medical personnel, and had to create institutions and services rapidly in many fields. Mental health was not isolated from this reality; it carried the same pressures as a young public-health system, often more intensely because of stigma and a small professional workforce.

Cultural diversity also shaped clinical encounters. Behavior that appeared unusual or suspicious to staff could carry a different meaning within another culture, language, or family tradition. When professional and patient do not share a language or cultural framework, silence can more easily be interpreted as noncooperation, an unfamiliar belief as a delusion, or resistance as dangerousness. This challenge is not unique to Israel, but in a society of rapid immigration it acquired particular importance. The question of rights therefore begins before the decision to hospitalize: it begins with the ability to understand the person standing before you.

The family held a dual role. On one hand, it was often the main source of information, care, and supervision, especially when community services were limited. On the other hand, family power could strongly affect a person's path - who would be brought for examination, who would remain at home, and who would be referred to an institution. In a reality without a rich range of alternatives, families sometimes had to choose among difficult options, and it was not always clear where concern ended and control began.

Israel's security reality added another layer to the mental-health system over the years. Periods of war, terrorism, and population displacement increase distress and bring psychiatric services into contact with people who were not previously part of the system. They can also blur the boundary between a human response to extreme circumstances and a disorder requiring medical treatment. The ability to distinguish between the two, and to offer support without rushing to turn every form of distress into a diagnosis, is part of the maturity of a mental-health system in a society living under continuing strain.

Early Israeli history therefore teaches a lesson that remains important today: law does not operate in a vacuum. The same legal authority can have a different meaning in an overloaded system, in a multicultural society, and during a period in which alternatives to hospitalization are scarce. To understand the first law, it must be read within the reality in which it was enacted, not only through contemporary concepts.

The Israeli mental-health story is inseparable from the story of the state. Waves of immigration, wars, poverty, construction of a new health system, and shortages of professionals placed heavy pressures on institutions already limited in resources. People arrived with different languages, traditions, and explanations of distress. What appeared to medical staff as unusual behavior could carry another meaning within a community, family, or culture unfamiliar to the clinicians.

The cultural gap is especially important in psychiatry because diagnosis depends heavily on conversation, behavior, and context. In physical medicine, it is sometimes possible to rely on a blood test or imaging; in mental health, words and their meanings occupy a central place. Where there is no shared language, the risk of misunderstanding increases. The history of the system is therefore also a history of translation - not only between languages but between understandings of family, religion, shame, responsibility, and treatment.

In the state's early years, when resources were limited and the institutional model still dominated internationally, it is understandable that care centered on hospitals. Yet that choice created a path that influenced the following decades: budgets, personnel, and knowledge were built around institutions, and only gradually did the center of gravity move to the community. The 1955 law would emerge from this reality - as a law intended to regulate an existing system, not to redesign it from the ground up.

Local history also shows how deeply a medical institution is influenced by the society around it. During periods of security tension, mass immigration, or economic distress, the mental-health system must respond not only to illness in a narrow sense but also to the effects of trauma, loss, and disruption of life structures. When an entire society is occupied with survival and institution-building, the right to choose a therapist or receive services close to home is not always at the top of the agenda. In retrospect it is easy to identify what was missing; at the time, the system operated within severe constraints.

Precisely for that reason, it is important to distinguish explanation from justification. The fact that a young state operated under scarcity does not make every impairment of rights inevitable, but it helps explain why a centralized institutional model took root. History allows us to understand choices without turning them into permanent norms. When conditions change, arrangements should change as well.

That lesson remains relevant. A service created as a temporary response to crisis can over time become a permanent structure simply because the system becomes accustomed to working that way. A health system should therefore periodically ask not only whether a service functions, but whether the reason for which it was built still exists. The history of mental health in Israel is to a large extent a story of moving from solutions born of immediate necessity to a system that now seeks to justify itself in terms of quality, equality, and rights.

The law enacted in 1955 expressed these assumptions. It was a significant step in regulating the field, but it also reflected the limits of the rights discourse of its time. Four decades later, those limits would become one of the reasons for replacing it.

Chapter Eleven

Treatment of Mental Patients Law, 1955

Israel's First Law in the Field

The Treatment of Mental Patients Law, 5715-1955, was published on July 6, 1955. It was the first Israeli law dedicated specifically to regulating the treatment of people with mental illness and the conditions and powers relating to their hospitalization. The very enactment of legislation was important: it replaced a situation in which such a sensitive field rested largely on prior arrangements and administrative powers, and established an explicit Israeli framework.

Read from today's perspective, however, the law reveals the difference between two conceptions. One is regulation: the state cannot leave psychiatric hospitalization without rules. The other is rights: what rules are necessary to protect a person against arbitrary deprivation of liberty? The 1955 law advanced considerably in the first dimension but was more limited in the second.

In the Knesset debate, Health Minister Yosef Serlin emphasized a desire to avoid, as far as possible, a judicial process that would frighten the person or relatives and make treatment resemble the prison system. This position also arose from a wish to reduce stigma. If psychiatric hospitalization is medical treatment, the underlying argument was, there is no need to turn every admission into an adversarial proceeding between the state and the individual.

There is a humane element in that reasoning. A person in crisis does not necessarily need a courtroom, and legal confrontation can intensify fear and mistrust. The difficulty appears when hospitalization is involuntary. Once the door is locked and the person is not free to leave, the relationship is no longer solely medical. The state is exercising real governmental power.

One of the important lessons in the development of the law follows from this point: it is possible to preserve a humane and nonthreatening procedure while still guaranteeing independent review. The assumption that one must choose between 'treatment' and 'law' proved incomplete. In a field where treatment can include deprivation of liberty, procedural rights are part of fair treatment rather than something external to it.

The 1955 law gave a central role to the medical system and district psychiatry. The mechanism for involuntary hospitalization relied to a considerable extent on professional judgment. This reflected the paternalistic medicine of the period, in which the physician was regarded not only as an expert in diagnosis and treatment but at times also as the person authorized to determine the patient's best interests.

The problem is not reliance on expertise itself. Questions of psychiatric hospitalization cannot be decided without clinical assessment. The problem arises when clinical expertise becomes, by itself, the source of authority to deprive liberty, and when safeguards are too weak or arrive too late.

That gap became clearer over the years. During the 1980s, in efforts to amend the law, criticism was raised that involuntary hospitalization ordered by the district psychiatrist was not automatically limited to a short period followed by mandatory external review. The very need for such amendments shows how the conception of procedure had changed: what had once appeared to be therapeutic flexibility increasingly came to be seen as a risk to liberty.

Hospitalization as Treatment and as Governmental Power

To understand the law, two truths must be held at the same time. First, there are acute psychiatric conditions in which rapid intervention may prevent serious harm and save lives. Second, psychiatric diagnosis alone should not turn a person into an exception to ordinary rights.

The old law had difficulty sharply separating these truths. Institutional structures and medical culture gave hospitalization a central status. In such a system, questions that now appear essential - Is there a less restrictive alternative? Is the risk concrete? Does the person understand the procedure? Can the person make a case before an independent body? - were not always at the center.

Historically, this was not unique to Israel. In many countries, mental-health laws were initially organized around powers of admission and detention and only later around rights, due process, and review. Israel was part of the same international trajectory.

It would be wrong to portray the 1955 law as legislation entirely indifferent to the possibility of harm. Even when it was introduced, concern was expressed about malicious hospitalization, for example in order to seize a person's property. The law sought to create protections in this respect, and the legislature recognized that the power to hospitalize could be abused.

That recognition is important in principle. It shows that even in the 1950s it was understood that psychiatric hospitalization was not a neutral act. The ability to define someone as requiring hospitalization could affect property, status, family, and reputation. Yet the safeguards focused largely on preventing obvious malicious abuse, and less on the broader question of whether a decision made in good faith might still impair rights disproportionately.

This is a fundamental distinction. A modern rights-based system does not ask only whether the decision maker acted maliciously. It also asks whether the decision was necessary, whether it was supported by evidence, whether a less harmful alternative existed, and whether the person had an effective opportunity to present his or her position.

The language of the law also reflects its period. The Hebrew term traditionally rendered as 'mental patient' was a natural part of medical and legal discourse and remains in the title of the 1991 law and in parts of its wording. Yet such terminology is not merely linguistic. It can blur the distinction between the person and the diagnosis and turn a medical condition into a total identity.

Legal language creates reality. When a law defines a group of people through illness, it can reinforce the sense that they form a separate category of citizens. This is one reason contemporary professional and public discourse increasingly uses language that places the person before the diagnosis.

This book uses historical terminology where it is necessary to understand the law, but does not adopt that language as a comprehensive description of people.

Four Decades of Change Begin

The 1955 law remained in force, with amendments and changes, for more than thirty-five years. During that period, the world around it changed. Psychiatry changed; new medications enabled some people to live outside institutions; criticism of prolonged hospitalization developed; constitutional and administrative law grew stronger; and other countries increased oversight of civil deprivation of liberty.

Within Israel, gaps gradually became visible between a law built in a relatively institutional and paternalistic world and a newer conception that gave greater weight to the person's will and to scrutiny of state power. The result was not immediate replacement. Legal change in a field this sensitive usually advances in layers: amendment, criticism, professional debate, judicial interpretation, a new proposal - and only then a new law.

Reading the 1955 law with contemporary eyes may create a sense of great distance, but it is worth remembering that the law itself was part of a movement toward regulation. It sought to move weighty decisions out of a gray zone and into a framework of authority, responsibility, and documentation. The very existence of dedicated legislation signaled that the state recognized psychiatric hospitalization not as a private act between physician and patient but as an exercise of power requiring rules.

The rules, however, reflected the hierarchy of the period. The physician and the system stood at the center; the individual's voice was weaker, and the family was sometimes viewed as a natural intermediary between the person and the institution. Questions now taken for granted - what was explained to the patient, whether the person was represented, how an appeal could be made, whether a less restrictive alternative existed - did not carry the same weight. This was not only a matter of wording. It reflected a medical culture in which professional authority was itself regarded as a central source of legitimacy.

The terms used by the law matter as well. Legal language is not neutral; it reveals how an era views the people to whom the law applies. When a person is defined first and foremost by illness, it becomes easier for legal identity to shrink to clinical status. The later shift in discourse - from a person who 'is mentally ill' to a citizen, patient, or person living with a mental-health condition - is more than linguistic. It changes the starting point: do we describe the person by the diagnosis, or do we describe a medical condition as one part of the life of a person who has rights?

In this sense, the 1955 law is a historical document that allows us to see how the relationship between treatment and liberty was constructed in the young state. It was not an extreme anomaly compared with the world of its time, which is precisely why it is important. It shows that paternalism did not arise from malice but from a broad institutional belief that the person who knows what is best for the patient may also decide on the patient's behalf. Only when that assumption began to crack did the need for a new law emerge.

The nature of the law can also be understood through what is absent from it from a contemporary perspective. A modern reader almost automatically looks for provisions on consent, representation, information, community alternatives, and rapid review. The very expectation reveals how much legal culture has changed. In the 1950s, the regulatory focus was primarily on who was authorized to act and how the system would operate. Today, we expect a law dealing with deprivation of liberty to answer, in the same breath, what rights belong to the person against whom the power is exercised.

The gap is therefore not merely between an old law and a new law but between two different ideas about the function of legislation. The first sees law as an instrument that organizes powers; the second sees it also as an instrument that protects the individual from organized power. Viewed in this way, the reason the 1955 law could not ultimately be modernized through technical changes alone becomes clearer. A change in perspective itself was required.

The 1955 law is important not only for its provisions but because it reflects how a young state understood the relationship between medicine and authority. The legislature sought to create order in a field where major decisions were sometimes made without a uniform framework. The enactment itself was a step toward the rule of law: it defined offices and powers rather than leaving decisions solely to institutional custom. Yet the language and balances of the law carried the worldview of the period, in which protection of the person and the public received greater weight than the person's participation in the decision.

This gap was not unique to Israel. Many laws enacted in the middle of the twentieth century rested on the assumption that physicians and administrators were the actors who knew what was required, while the patient's role was more limited. Procedural rights as they are understood today - representation, rapid review, accessible explanation, participation, and decision-making support - were not yet central. It is therefore not useful to judge the law only by the standard of 2026. It is more important to understand how the conception changed and why a framework that seemed reasonable to its contemporaries gradually became inadequate.

The accumulation of criticism over the years illustrates a familiar legal process. A law does not become obsolete in a single day. Difficult cases emerge first; interpretations then attempt to reduce harm; later, the gap between the text and new values grows. At a certain point, local amendments are no longer enough. This is how the ground was prepared for the 1991 law - not as a revolution that appeared in an instant, but as the result of decades during which the system, society, and law changed around an aging statute.

The 1955 law is therefore more than an old chapter in the statute book. It is a point of reference that makes it possible to understand the significance of the 1991 law. Without knowing how much authority the system once possessed, it is difficult to evaluate what changed and what remained similar.

Chapter Twelve

Four Decades of Change

Psychiatry Changes, and the Law Must Change with It

Between 1955 and 1991, developments in Israel and around the world fundamentally changed the debate over mental health. This was not the result of a single event. Several processes unfolded in parallel: advances in medication, a gradual decline in dependence on long-term hospitalization, the development of community-based services, criticism of institutions, the strengthening of administrative law, and the growing status of human rights.

When a law is enacted, it fixes within its text many of the assumptions of its time. The 1955 law assumed that psychiatric institutions were a central axis of treatment and that broad medical authority was a reasonable means of managing severe conditions. As reality changed, the gap between the assumptions embedded in the law and the new possibilities became increasingly visible.

The introduction of antipsychotic medications and other psychiatric drugs did not eliminate the need for hospitalization, nor did it solve all the problems associated with severe mental illness. It did, however, expand the possibility of treating some people outside institutions and of reducing prolonged hospital stays. This development created a new legal question: if a therapeutic objective can be achieved by a less restrictive means, is it still justified to keep a person in hospital? This question is an early expression of the principle of proportionality.

The right to liberty does not require the state to refrain from every form of coercion, but it does require the state to consider whether the same objective can be achieved through a measure that causes less harm.

The shift toward community care also changed the meaning of discharge. It was once possible to regard discharge as the end of treatment. Gradually, it became clear that discharge without housing, employment, outpatient care, family support, and continuity of treatment can produce a revolving door of crisis, hospitalization, and repeated discharge.

International criticism of psychiatric hospitals also reached Israel. A closed institution can provide protection and treatment, but it can also create dependency, isolation, and loss of everyday skills. The longer hospitalization continues, the more pressing the question becomes: is the person still there because intensive medical care is necessary, or because no suitable alternative exists in the community?

This distinction is critical. If a person remains in hospital because supported housing or rehabilitation services are unavailable, the deprivation of liberty does not arise only from the person's medical condition. It also reflects the structure of services that the state has chosen to fund.

From this emerged a principle that would later become central: the right to liberty is protected not only by restricting the power to hospitalize. It also depends on investment in alternatives that make it possible for people to live outside hospital.

At the same time, the law itself was changing. A decision by a district psychiatrist is not merely a medical decision; it is a decision of a public authority with profound consequences for a person's liberty. As Israeli law developed a stronger conception of review over administrative authorities, so too did the demand grow that psychiatric decisions be reasoned, evidence-based, and limited.

Amendments debated during the 1980s illustrate this process. One criticism was that involuntary hospitalization under the old law was not automatically subject to a short and clearly defined period at the end of which independent review was required. The idea that a person could remain hospitalized until the system itself decided to release them increasingly appeared inadequate.

The need for review does not express blanket distrust of psychiatrists. It expresses a democratic principle: the person who recommends deprivation of liberty should not also be the only person who decides whether that deprivation will continue.

General medicine was changing as well. The model in which the physician decided and the patient complied gradually lost its exclusive status. The concept of informed consent grew stronger, together with recognition that a person may choose differently from what the physician would choose on that person's behalf.

In psychiatry, the transition is more complex because the illness itself may, in some situations, impair judgment or the perception of reality. Complexity, however, is not a reason to abandon the principle. On the contrary, it requires a more precise examination of when decision-making ability is actually impaired and when the person is simply making a choice with which professionals disagree.

This distinction is particularly important. A person does not lose the right to autonomy merely because a mental disorder has been diagnosed. Even during hospitalization, and even in crisis, there may be many decisions that the person remains capable of making. A binary view of 'capable' or 'incapable' misses the fact that decision-making ability may depend on the subject, the moment, and the support available to the person.

By the late 1980s and early 1990s, the need to replace the law had matured. The explanatory materials for the new bill stated this explicitly: the proposed law was intended to replace the 1955 law on the basis of experience accumulated in its implementation, advances in psychiatric treatment, and the new approach of directing resources toward medical treatment in the community.

That formulation is important because it shows that the new law was not born solely from legal criticism. It was also connected to a change in clinical and system-wide thinking. If community treatment was becoming an objective, the mechanisms of hospitalization, discharge, and involuntary treatment had to be adapted accordingly.

The bill underwent extended discussion in the Knesset Labor and Welfare Committee. Representatives of the Ministry of Health, psychiatrists, lawyers, and other professionals participated in the deliberations. The detailed parliamentary discussion itself reflected a change in the status of the issue: involuntary hospitalization was no longer regarded only as an internal professional matter for the health system, but as a public and legal question.

1991: A New Law, but Not the End of the Dispute

The Treatment of Mental Patients Law, 5751-1991, was published in January 1991 and entered into force on April 8, 1991, ninety days after publication. On that date it replaced the 1955 law. It created more detailed mechanisms for compulsory examination, involuntary hospitalization, compulsory outpatient treatment, psychiatric review committees, and appeals. In this respect, it strengthened both regulation and oversight.

Yet 1991 should not be described as the completion of the transition from paternalism to rights. The law itself preceded Basic Law: Human Dignity and Liberty, the Patients' Rights Law, the Equal Rights for Persons with Disabilities Law, the community rehabilitation law, and the Convention on the Rights of Persons with Disabilities. In other words, it was enacted immediately before another major Israeli and international wave of rights development.

The change from the 1950s to the 1990s also occurred in public consciousness. More people encountered mental-health services outside closed institutions, more families demanded explanations, and both the media and the courts increasingly addressed not only whether treatment had been provided but also the quality of conditions and the manner in which authority was exercised. As Israeli society became more legally conscious, a medical decision that affected liberty could no longer remain an internal professional matter.

Medicine changed as well. Pharmacological and community-based treatment made it possible in many cases to shorten hospital stays and manage conditions that previously would have led to prolonged institutionalization. When a practical alternative exists, it becomes more difficult to justify deprivation of liberty simply because that was the customary practice in the past. Medical technology, organizational change, and human rights worked together here: each weakened, to some extent, the assumption that the hospital was the natural destination for every severe crisis.

The transition, however, was not abrupt. Different outlooks coexisted within the same system. A professional might see themselves as protecting a patient while resisting outside oversight that seemed to interfere with clinical work. A family might demand stronger rights for a relative and, at the same time, ask the state to hospitalize that person out of fear for their life. A person might resist hospitalization with all their strength and later say that it saved them. This reality helps explain why legal change in this field cannot be built on a simple story of 'the system versus the patient.'

The new law therefore had to do two almost contradictory things: preserve the state's ability to intervene in extreme situations while making the use of that power exceptional, reasoned, and subject to review. The difficulty was not resolved in 1991. It was given a more advanced framework within which it continues to be negotiated to this day.

The change between 1955 and 1991 occurred not only in the statute book. It took place in hospital wards, universities, courts, and public discourse. New medications allowed some hospital stays to be shortened, ideas of community care became stronger, and rights-based law began to demand reasons and review in areas that had once depended almost entirely on professional judgment. None of these processes would have been sufficient on its own; together they changed what society expected from the law.

Israeli society changed as well. The individual gradually gained a more central place in relation to institutions, while questions of information, consent, and professional accountability became more prominent in health care. Psychiatry could not remain outside that movement. If hospitalization had once been treated as evidence that the physician knew what was best for the person, it became increasingly clear that a decision to deprive someone of liberty must also be capable of explanation to those outside the medical system.

This period also demonstrates how much legal reform depends on the accumulation of cultural change. A new law can accelerate a process, but it is difficult for legislation alone to create an entirely new outlook. When professionals, families, judges, and patients are already beginning to ask different questions, the law becomes a framework that gathers those changes together. The 1991 law is therefore better understood not as a starting point but as a point of convergence: an attempt to translate into legal principles a reality that no longer fit the world of 1955.

The path to a new law is also shaped by the way institutions learn from cases. An unusual incident that reaches a court, a family complaint, criticism by a public body, or a professional debate can expose a gap with which the system has learned to live. Not every case produces an amendment, but their accumulation changes the boundary of what is considered reasonable. What was once simply 'the way things are done' gradually becomes a practice that demands an explanation.

This is how a culture of review develops. At first, professionals may experience legal intervention as a threat to their authority. Over time, some of the rules become part of professional practice itself: good documentation, explanation, peer review, and time limits. The boundary between 'law' and 'medicine' becomes less sharp because protection of rights is incorporated into the standard of care.

Public language changes as well. Once concepts such as autonomy, informed consent, and dignity become familiar in general medicine, it becomes difficult to justify a system in which they stop at the entrance to a psychiatric ward. Psychiatry is therefore shaped by broader social developments. The 1991 law would express the shift but would not complete it; on the contrary, shortly after its enactment Israel entered a new constitutional era that would raise further questions that had not stood at the center of the original drafting process.

The 1991 law is therefore, in many respects, a transitional law. It sought to limit and structure coercion while still accepting coercion as a central part of the system's toolkit. That tension lies at the heart of the next chapter.

Chapter Thirteen

Treatment of Mental Patients Law, 1991: Major Change, Partial Revolution

A New Law for a Changing World

The Treatment of Mental Patients Law, 5751-1991, was published on January 8, 1991. According to the legislative record, the bill originated as a private member's initiative by Knesset Member Shoshana Arbeli-Almozlino, and the parliamentary process was accompanied by extensive professional discussion. Section 49 provided that the law would enter into force ninety days after publication, and it therefore took effect on April 8, 1991. On that date it replaced the 1955 law and became the principal statutory framework that continues to regulate involuntary psychiatric examination and hospitalization in Israel, alongside hospitalization and treatment ordered by courts and other arrangements.

Historically, the law marked clear progress. It was more detailed than its predecessor, established conditions and powers, created mechanisms of appeal and oversight, and recognized that deprivation of liberty requires procedure. At the same time, it was not a rights statute in the modern sense of the term. Its central purpose was to regulate treatment and coercion, not to eliminate the distinct legal framework separating psychiatry from ordinary medical treatment.

One of the law's important principles is that the mere existence of mental illness is not enough to justify compulsory examination or involuntary hospitalization. The coercive provisions depend on additional conditions, including a substantial impairment of judgment or reality testing as a consequence of the illness, together with elements of risk or serious harm, depending on the particular legal route.

This principle is important from a human-rights perspective. A diagnosis is a medical description; it is not a license to deprive a person of liberty. Two people with the same diagnosis may be in entirely different positions in terms of functioning, risk, and decision-making ability.

Israeli case law has also clarified over time that the concept of 'mental illness' may not be interpreted without limits. Where the law permits coercion on the basis of illness, there must be a real connection between the mental condition and the impairment of judgment or reality testing, and between those impairments and the danger or serious harm on which the proposed exercise of authority is based.

In many cases, compulsory hospitalization is preceded by a psychiatric examination. The law distinguishes between urgent and non-urgent routes. Under the urgent route, the statutory basis includes, among other things, circumstances in which the person's condition creates an immediate physical danger to self or others, together with the law's other requirements and refusal to undergo examination.

The non-urgent route permits intervention where the danger is not immediate and in additional circumstances enumerated by the law, such as severe impairment of the ability to care for basic needs, causing another person severe psychological suffering in a manner that seriously disrupts that person's life, or serious damage to property - all subject to the statutory conditions and to a connection between the mental state and the relevant conduct.

The distinction between urgent and non-urgent procedures is not merely technical. It expresses the principle of proportionality: the more immediate the risk, the more rapidly the state may be permitted to act. Where there is no urgency, there is correspondingly more room for procedure, additional examination, and consideration of alternatives.

Involuntary Hospitalization: Deprivation of Liberty in the Name of Treatment and Protection

Involuntary hospitalization is the most serious intervention the law permits in the ordinary civil process. A person who does not wish to remain in hospital is required to stay there and, at times, to receive treatment within a setting from which departure is restricted. The justification therefore cannot be reduced to the claim that treatment is 'recommended.'

The law constructs authority around a combination of mental condition, impairment of judgment or reality testing, and conditions involving dangerousness or serious harm. In this way, it seeks to distinguish between a person who needs help but remains entitled to refuse it and a situation in which the state concludes that nonintervention would create danger or serious harm sufficient to justify deprivation of liberty.

Even this structure does not resolve every difficulty. Risk assessment is not an exact science. It rests on clinical information, history, behavior, circumstances, and signs that may be interpreted in different ways. An error in one direction may result in harm to the person or to others; an error in the other may result in the confinement of someone whose liberty did not need to be taken away.

The law must therefore operate within uncertainty. The answer is not to pretend that the future can be predicted with certainty, but to require a factual basis, causal connection, reasons, proportionality, and repeated review.

One of the important changes from the older approach is that involuntary hospitalization is not supposed to be a one-time decision of indefinite duration. The law establishes limited periods and mechanisms for extension and review. The logic is clear: mental states change. A justification that existed on the first day may no longer exist two weeks or two months later.

Repeated review should be substantive rather than ceremonial. The question is not merely whether the diagnosis remains, but whether the conditions that justify deprivation of liberty still exist and whether a less restrictive alternative is available.

This principle connects law and treatment. Therapeutic success may itself weaken the justification for continued coercion. A system that continues to hold a person only because hospitalization benefits them turns medical success into a reason to continue depriving them of liberty - a result that is difficult to justify from a rights perspective.

The law establishes district psychiatric committees whose functions include decisions concerning continued hospitalization and appeals. In their current form, the committees combine a legal member with psychiatrists. The composition reflects recognition that a decision about involuntary hospitalization cannot be purely medical. Psychiatrists contribute clinical expertise; the legal member is intended to bring the perspective of law, evidence, and procedure. The combination is meant to create an equilibrium between two worlds.

In practice, the committee's independence and the effectiveness of review depend not only on composition but on the culture of the hearing: does the person receive a genuine opportunity to speak? Are alternatives examined? Are the reasons individualized? Is there willingness to disagree with the treating team's position?

Effective review does not require the committee frequently to reject the hospital's recommendation. The rate of acceptance or rejection is not, by itself, a measure of quality. The real measure is whether each case is reconsidered rather than merely stamped with approval after the decision has already been made.

The Right of Appeal and Legal Representation

The ability to challenge an order of hospitalization or a decision to continue it is a basic component of due process. A person whose liberty has been taken away should know why, where an appeal may be filed, and within what time. In the modern system there is also a right to state-funded legal representation in proceedings concerning involuntary hospitalization and compulsory treatment, and the system is required to inform the person of that right.

Representation changes the balance of power. The hospital possesses the medical record, the professionals, and the clinical language. The hospitalized person may be in crisis, under medication, and in an unfamiliar environment. Without assistance, it is difficult to expect that person to formulate a legal argument, request relevant material, or identify a suitable alternative.

The lawyer is not a psychiatrist and does not replace clinical judgment. The lawyer's role is to ensure that power has been exercised lawfully and that the person's voice is not swallowed by the professional process.

The law also permits compulsory outpatient treatment. At first glance, this appears less intrusive than hospitalization: the person remains in the community rather than behind a locked ward door. In appropriate cases, it is indeed an alternative that restricts physical liberty less severely.

Yet 'less intrusive' does not mean 'free of coercion.' When continued liberty in the community is conditioned on compliance with treatment instructions, governmental power remains present. The person knows that refusal can lead to further proceedings and even hospitalization. Compulsory outpatient treatment therefore raises its own questions: how much real choice exists? Are alternatives available? Does coercion improve continuity of care or weaken trust? Where is the boundary between therapeutic supervision and control over everyday life?

These questions become central in international comparison because different countries have adopted different models of community treatment orders.

The historical irony is that the Treatment of Mental Patients Law was enacted immediately before a major constitutional change in Israel. In 1992, Basic Law: Human Dignity and

Liberty was enacted. The liberty of the individual, bodily integrity, and human dignity suddenly received stronger and more explicit constitutional status.

From that point onward, the 1991 law had to be read within a new normative world. The question was no longer only whether the district psychiatrist had acted within the empowering section, but also whether the infringement of liberty pursued a proper purpose and went no further than necessary.

The Ministry of Health itself notes that legal developments after 1991 required the law to be interpreted and applied in light of Basic Law: Human Dignity and Liberty and additional legislation. This completed the point of transition: the 1991 law did not remain frozen as it had been on the day of enactment; a new layer of rights grew around it and changed how coercive powers had to be understood.

Achievements and Limits of the Law

The 1991 law was an important step. It improved regulation, strengthened oversight mechanisms, established procedures and time limits, and made clear that coercive authority is not unlimited. That progress should not be underestimated.

Yet it remains a law centered on regulating the circumstances in which the state may intervene against a person's wishes. Its language, institutions, and structure were created before the patients' rights revolution, before equality legislation for persons with disabilities, before the community rehabilitation law, and before the United Nations Convention on the Rights of Persons with Disabilities.

The important question, therefore, is not whether the law was progressive in 1991. It is whether it still adequately expresses the rights conception of the twenty-first century. To answer that question, we must turn to the next wave of legislation: human dignity, informed consent, equality, rehabilitation, and life in the community. This is where the broader Israeli rights revolution begins.

The meaning of the law becomes clearer if we think about the path a person actually travels. A crisis does not begin in a statutory section. It begins at home, at work, in the street, or in a clinic. Family members may spend days trying to persuade a person to accept help; police or medical staff may become involved; a person may arrive voluntarily at an emergency department and later ask to leave. Only at some point does formal authority enter the picture.

For the person, this entire sequence may be experienced as one event. For the law, it consists of a series of separate decisions, each of which requires its own legal basis.

From the patient's perspective, however, the system is not fragmented at all. The person does not necessarily know the difference between a district psychiatrist's decision, a department director's decision, the treating physician's recommendation, and the committee's decision. All of them may be experienced simply as 'the system.' That is why a simple and continuous explanation matters: who decided what, for how long, who can change the decision, and what happens next. Without such an explanation, even a sophisticated legal mechanism may feel like a chain of orders over which the person has no influence.

The gap between institutional complexity and the simplicity of human experience appears in many public systems, but it is particularly acute in psychiatry because the person may at that moment be frightened, suspicious, or overwhelmed. Procedural rights must therefore be translated into language that can be used in real time, rather than remaining knowledge that belongs only to lawyers.

This institutional division matters because it enables review. The person who ordered an examination is not necessarily the person who decides on continued hospitalization; the treating team is not the only body that examines the lawfulness of detention; and a decision that appeared justified on the first day must be tested again when the person's condition changes. Protection is built through multiple decision points. They cannot guarantee the absence of error, but they recognize that authority this powerful should neither be concentrated in one person nor continue simply through inertia.

Procedure, however, can become a ritual if it is not carried out meaningfully. A committee does not protect rights merely because it exists; it must genuinely hear the person, examine documents, question the team, and be capable of reaching a different conclusion. Legal representation has little value if counsel meets the person only a few minutes before the hearing. An explanation of rights is insufficient if it is given when the person cannot understand it and is never repeated once the condition stabilizes.

To understand the meaning of the 1991 law, it is useful to imagine the moment at which the statute meets a person rather than a section. Someone is brought for examination against their wishes. From the system's perspective, a route of powers, conditions, deadlines, and appeals begins; from the person's perspective, a personal event begins in which they want to know who decided, why, for how long, and what can be done about it. The quality of the law is tested where these two descriptions meet. A good legal framework must be precise enough for decision makers and clear enough for the person on whom the decision is imposed.

The new law created more meaningful mechanisms of review, but it did not eliminate the basic tension. Even a law with committees and appeals grants the state exceptional power. The question is therefore not only whether review exists, but whether it arrives in time, whether the person can participate, and whether the reviewing body feels free to disagree with the clinical assessment. A review mechanism that becomes ceremonial loses much of its purpose; one that forces the decision to be reasoned anew actually changes the balance of power.

It is also important to recognize what the law could not have anticipated. It was enacted before the informed-consent revolution of the Patients' Rights Law, before equality legislation, before the rehabilitation law, and before the development of supported decision-making. Some of today's tension therefore does not necessarily arise from a flaw that was obvious in 1991, but from the fact that the surrounding normative environment has changed. The law stayed in place while the legal order around it moved forward. That gap will become central when we return to the law at the end of the book and ask whether the framework can continue to be updated or whether a new structure is required.

This is both the limit and the strength of the 1991 law. It created a structure in which coercion was no longer merely an internal medical act, but a decision that had to exist within a legal framework. Yet it was still written in a world in which the very existence of a separate legal system for involuntary psychiatric hospitalization was taken for granted. The developments that followed would begin to challenge even that starting point.

Part Five

The Rights Revolution in Israel

Chapter Fourteen

Human Dignity, Autonomy, and Informed Consent

1992: Liberty Acquires Constitutional Status

Only one year after the Treatment of Mental Patients Law was enacted, Israel adopted Basic Law: Human Dignity and Liberty. Published on March 25, 1992, it gave explicit constitutional status to a series of rights, including life, bodily integrity, dignity, property, personal liberty, and privacy. For mental health, the implications were especially profound: involuntary hospitalization was no longer simply the exercise of a statutory power; it was an infringement of a constitutional right to liberty that had to be interpreted and exercised narrowly, for a proper purpose, and to no greater extent than necessary.

The Basic Law did not repeal the Treatment of Mental Patients Law, nor did it declare every involuntary hospitalization unlawful. The change was different: the normative starting point became stronger. When the state deprives a person of liberty, it must justify the infringement. The question is no longer only 'Does the law permit this?' but also 'How should that permission be interpreted so as to respect the person as fully as possible?'

This represents a change in legal culture. Medical authority remains essential, but it does not operate outside constitutional discourse. Even a decision aimed at treatment and protection may be excessively intrusive if it is broader than necessary.

It is easy to speak of 'human dignity' in general terms. In psychiatric hospitalization, dignity takes a very concrete form: is the person addressed by name? Is the reason for hospitalization explained? Is privacy protected? Are clothes and personal belongings taken without need? Can the person contact family members and a lawyer? Do staff speak about the person in their presence as though they were not there? Is the person's position heard even when it is not accepted?

Dignity does not eliminate the need for treatment. It changes the manner in which treatment is delivered. The same medical intervention can be carried out in two entirely different ways from the standpoint of human experience. A rights-based system does not ask only whether the staff acted 'for the patient's benefit.' It also asks whether the person remains a subject with a voice throughout the process.

This is especially important in psychiatry because diagnosis can quickly become a filter through which every statement by the person is interpreted as a symptom. Anger about hospitalization may be labeled agitation; suspicion of staff may be interpreted as part of the illness; insistence on discharge may be seen as lack of insight. Sometimes those interpretations are clinically accurate. But when every protest becomes proof that the protester should not be heard, a self-reinforcing circle is created that weakens the possibility of criticism.

The Patients' Rights Law, 5756-1996, deepened the move from paternalistic medicine toward medicine that recognizes autonomy. Its purpose is to establish the rights of people who seek or receive medical treatment and to protect their dignity and privacy. At its center stands the principle of informed consent: as a general rule, medical treatment should not be given without the patient's consent after the information necessary for the decision has been provided.

Informed consent is not a signature on a form. It is a process of information and understanding: the diagnosis, the prospects and risks, the nature of the treatment, its expected benefit, side effects, available alternatives, and the option of not receiving treatment. The law requires information to be provided in a manner that allows the patient the greatest possible degree of understanding and voluntary choice.

This conception changes the balance of power. The physician brings professional knowledge; the patient brings their life, values, preferences, and priorities. A good medical decision is not simply the decision that maximizes a clinical outcome according to the team's measures. It is a decision that fits, as far as possible, the person whose body and life are at stake.

And What Happens in Psychiatry?

Here the tension becomes sharper. The Patients' Rights Law creates a broad rule of consent, while the Treatment of Mental Patients Law establishes special pathways that, in certain circumstances, permit treatment and hospitalization without consent. Psychiatry therefore exists within the system of patients' rights but also within an exceptional arrangement that permits departure from the general rule.

The exception should not swallow the rule. The fact that a person has been hospitalized involuntarily does not mean that every medical decision in that person's life may thereafter be made without their wishes. Even within involuntary hospitalization there remains room for explanation, for choice among alternatives, for consent wherever possible, and for distinguishing treatment that may lawfully be imposed from other decisions in which the person's own will remains decisive.

This point matters because institutional systems can easily create a kind of 'contagion' of lost autonomy. One decision to hospitalize a person without consent can turn into a practical assumption that the patient has authority over nothing at all. A rights-based approach requires the opposite: the exception must be confined to its proper boundaries.

One of the most important distinctions in medicine is the difference between a decision with which professionals disagree and an inability to make a decision. A person may understand that a physician recommends a medication, understand the risks of refusing it, and still refuse because of side effects, past experience, personal values, or another preference.

If every refusal is automatically treated as evidence that the person 'does not understand their condition,' informed consent loses its meaning. Genuine consent exists only where there is a real possibility of saying no.

There are, on the other hand, situations in which an acute mental disorder can genuinely impair the ability to understand information, weigh consequences, or recognize reality. In those circumstances, law and medicine confront a difficult question: how can a person be protected without erasing that person as someone who has a will?

The modern answer increasingly moves away from automatic substitution of another person's will. It seeks accommodations, adapted explanations, time, a calm environment, and support for decision-making before concluding that the person cannot decide.

Psychiatric information is among the most sensitive information in the health system. Disclosure may affect employment, family relationships, insurance, licensing, and the way other people perceive the individual. Privacy is therefore not a technical appendix to care; it is part of the ability to seek treatment without fearing that treatment will become a public identity.

Even here, however, exceptions exist. In situations of danger or where the law requires disclosure, confidentiality is not absolute. The challenge is to prevent the exceptions from becoming routine. The information disclosed should be what is necessary, to the appropriate recipient, for the defined purpose - and no more.

An Unfinished Revolution

Basic Law: Human Dignity and Liberty and the Patients' Rights Law changed the legal language of medicine in Israel. They strengthened autonomy, privacy, and consent. The mental-health system, however, continued to operate under a special statute that permits coercion.

This created a normative tension that accompanies Israel to this day: how can a law that protects a patient's right to choose be reconciled with a law that, under certain conditions, permits that choice to be overridden?

Autonomy does not mean that a person always makes the 'right' decision. People refuse tests, persist in harmful habits, choose less effective treatment, and sometimes prefer quality of life to prolongation of life. In general medicine, we recognize that the right to choose includes the right to choose differently from the recommendation. Psychiatry is more complex because the disorder itself may impair judgment, insight, or the ability to understand the situation. But that is precisely where accuracy is required: impairment cannot automatically be inferred from the diagnosis.

Decision-making ability is decision-specific and time-specific. A person may struggle to understand a complex decision about property while knowing very clearly what treatment they are willing to receive; they may be confused in the morning and capable of a more coherent conversation in the evening. The question is therefore not whether the person is 'competent' in a general sense, but whether, at the particular moment, they can understand relevant information, weigh it, and communicate a choice. The more intrusive the decision, the greater the importance of an individualized assessment.

Autonomy itself does not exist in a vacuum. Most of us make decisions through conversations with partners, friends, physicians, or family members. Support does not contradict independence; at times it is a condition for it. A modern rights model therefore does not seek to leave a person alone in front of a consent form. It seeks to enable the person to receive information in an appropriate way, ask questions, consult others, and request time. The challenge is to make sure that support does not become substitution of someone else's will.

In practice, autonomy may be created in a very short conversation. A physician can say, 'This is the medication I recommend,' and stop there, or can add two questions: 'What worries you most about this treatment?' and 'What is most important for you to preserve in the coming period?' The answers may alter the choice between medications, the time of administration, or the pace of dose increases. This is not a surrender of expertise but a more accurate use of it. A medical recommendation becomes stronger when it understands the life into which it must fit.

In psychiatry, this distinction changes the point of view. Instead of asking only whether refusal may be overridden, the first question should be what is needed to enable the person to decide: must anxiety be reduced, must the explanation be given again, should someone the person trusts be brought in, should another option be offered, or can the decision safely wait? In this way autonomy becomes not merely an abstract principle but a therapeutic practice.

The Patients' Rights Law added to Israeli health care a language in which the patient is not merely the recipient of treatment but a person whose treatment is given with consent after information has been provided. In psychiatry, that language immediately encounters an exception: the Treatment of Mental Patients Law permits certain acts that do not depend on consent. This creates tension between a general law that places consent at the center and a special law that defines when departure from consent is permitted.

The way to address the tension is not to say that the special law 'cancels' autonomy. On the contrary, precisely where exceptional authority exists, everything that does not require the exception should remain within the sphere of choice. A person who is not free to leave a ward may still participate in choosing the time of a conversation, deciding who receives information, selecting among suitable medications, and planning discharge. Autonomy is therefore not an on-off switch but a space that may be narrowed only where justification exists.

Explanation itself is part of treatment. A patient who does not understand why a decision is being made against their wishes may experience it as arbitrary. Explanation does not guarantee agreement, and the person may continue to object. But explanation keeps the person within the conversation and makes clear that the system recognizes them as someone entitled to reasons. In crisis, explanations may need to be repeated. The right to information is not fulfilled by handing over a sheet of paper; it requires an effort to create understanding as far as possible.

Autonomy is tested most sharply when a person chooses differently from the professional recommendation. As long as the patient agrees, it is easy to say that choice is respected. The real test comes when the person prefers an option that the team regards as inferior. At that point, a distinction must be made between a decision the physician considers unwise and a decision the person is unable to make. Confusing the two is one of the principal sources of paternalism.

The distinction is not simple, because general medicine also includes situations in which illness affects understanding. Psychiatry, however, carries a particular risk: disagreement itself may be interpreted as part of the disorder. It is therefore important to examine the process of reasoning rather than the outcome alone. Does the person understand the information? Can they explain their reasons? Do they recognize the consequences even if they assign them different weight? Questions such as these respect the possibility that a person may make a choice different from the team's choice.

Autonomy does not guarantee that every decision will be safe. It guarantees that a person's entire life is not managed according to a single professional metric. Someone may prefer mental clarity to complete reduction of symptoms, privacy to family involvement, or less intensive treatment at the cost of some additional risk. As long as the law permits the choice and the person is capable of making it, medicine's role is to advise, not to substitute. Recognition of that boundary gives greater moral weight to the exceptional cases in which coercion may genuinely be justified.

The answer is not found in one statute. It is built from the combined effect of legislation, case law, ethics, and services. The next stage in the process moves from asking 'What may be done to a patient?' to asking 'How can a person with a disability be enabled to participate equally in society?'

Chapter Fifteen

Equal Rights for Persons with Disabilities

From Patient to Citizen

Until the 1990s, much of the legal discourse in mental health focused on what happened when a person entered the treatment system: hospitalization, examination, medication, and discharge. The Equal Rights for Persons with Disabilities Law, 5758-1998, widened the field of view. It asked what happens to the person outside the hospital - at work, in services, in public space, and in social life.

The law was published in March 1998 and entered into force at the beginning of 1999. Its principles are grounded in equality, dignity, and liberty, and its purpose is to enable a person with a disability to participate equally and actively in society, to achieve the greatest possible independence, and to enjoy privacy and dignity.

This is a profound shift. A person with a mental disorder is not only someone who may need treatment; the person is a citizen who should be able to work, study, use services, build a family, and make decisions about life.

The medical model focuses on impairment or illness: what is not functioning in the body or mind and how it can be treated. The social model asks a different question: what barriers in the environment turn difference into disability?

A person dealing with severe anxiety, for example, may experience genuine functional difficulty. Yet the degree of impairment in daily life also depends on the environment: does the workplace permit flexibility? Are public services accessible? Is stigma present? Is treatment available? Can an accommodation be obtained without disclosing more information than necessary?

The two models need not contradict one another. Medical treatment can be essential while society is simultaneously responsible for removing barriers. The problem arises when every difficulty is explained solely by the individual, thereby absolving the environment of any obligation to change.

Discrimination on the basis of mental health is not always stated openly. An employer does not necessarily say, 'I will not hire you because you have a mental disorder.' Exclusion may instead operate through assumptions: the person is regarded as unstable, dangerous, unpredictable, or less reliable.

This stigma is dangerous because it confuses diagnosis with functioning. Most people with a psychiatric diagnosis are not dangerous, and ability to work is not determined by the name of a diagnosis alone. An equal system must assess people according to their functioning and the actual requirements of a role, not according to generalized fear of a medical category.

The same principle applies in other areas. Questions concerning licensing, insurance, parenthood, or suitability for a framework should be based on a concrete and proportionate need, not on an assumption that a psychiatric history by itself negates ability.

Formal equality means giving everyone the same thing. Substantive equality recognizes that different people may need different tools in order to participate on an equal basis.

In mental health, an accommodation may involve flexibility in working hours during a period of treatment, providing information in a simpler form, accompaniment to a meeting, a quiet space, breaks, or a change in the way a service is delivered. Accommodations are not 'benefits' in the sense of charity. They are a way of removing a barrier that would otherwise deny participation.

The same logic later influences decision-making. If a person has difficulty understanding a complex document, the first question should not be whether someone else should be appointed to decide in their place, but whether the information can be adapted so that the person can decide for themselves.

Stigma as a Barrier to Rights

Legislation can prohibit discrimination, but it is much harder to legislate against a social image. Stigma acts before the courtroom: it affects whether a person seeks treatment, whether they disclose at work, their relationships, and the way they see themselves.

Self-stigma can be just as serious. A person who internalizes the message that mental illness makes them less capable may narrow their own aspirations. Genuine rehabilitation therefore requires more than providing a service; it also requires changing expectations - both the system's expectations and the person's own.

The major change brought by the equality law is the move from protective rights to rights of participation. It is not enough for the state simply to refrain from harm. It must create conditions in which a person can be part of society.

This principle lays the ground for the community rehabilitation law. If living in the community is a right rather than a prize for 'full recovery,' the state must develop housing, employment, education, and support that make such life possible.

This also generates a new criticism of prolonged hospitalization. If a person remains in an institution because no appropriate housing exists, the problem is not only medical. It is a problem of equality and resource allocation.

The complex test of equality in mental health often appears precisely when the disability is invisible. A person may arrive at work on time, speak fluently, and appear fully functional while investing enormous effort in coping with anxiety, mood fluctuations, concentration problems, or treatment side effects. When the difficulty is not visible, the environment may interpret it in moral terms: lack of seriousness, instability, laziness, or 'personality.' Discrimination can thus occur without any sign on the door; it takes place through the interpretation of behavior.

This leads to one of the most practical daily dilemmas: whether to disclose a mental-health condition in order to receive an accommodation. Disclosure can open the door to flexibility, understanding, and assistance. It can also change the way a manager, lecturer, or service provider treats the person. Someone who requests an accommodation may fear that from that moment every mistake will be attributed to the diagnosis. A genuine right to equality must therefore include protection of privacy and minimization of the information required. A person's medical history need not become an open file in order to consider a later start time, allow a break, provide written information, or schedule a meeting in a quieter environment.

The discussion of accommodations reveals the difference between identical treatment and fair treatment. A uniform rule may appear neutral while affecting people unequally. An employee required to arrive at a rigidly fixed hour after treatment that causes morning fatigue, a student sitting an examination in a crowded room after a period of severe anxiety, or a person required to retell their story at every station in a service system may all encounter barriers unrelated to their ability to perform the core task. When a small change removes the barrier without undermining the purpose of the service, the accommodation is not a privilege; it is how equality becomes practical.

Equality also has a less legal and more cultural dimension: the right to try. People emerging from crisis sometimes receive protective messages that narrow their options in advance: 'Do not take on too much,' 'It would be better to choose something simpler,' 'Perhaps you should not return to that kind of role.' Sometimes such advice arises from genuine concern, and sometimes it may be appropriate for a certain period. The problem begins when it becomes a permanent track determined by diagnosis. Protection against failure then becomes prevention of success.

The right to try also includes the right to make mistakes. A person without a mental disability may choose unsuitable work, leave a course of study, or change direction. If every setback by someone with a psychiatric history is treated as proof that the aspiration was 'unrealistic' from the outset, equality remains partial. An equal society does not guarantee success; it refrains from deciding in advance who is not entitled to compete for it.

Equality in mental health becomes especially sharp when an institutional decision is justified in the name of 'caution.' An employer, insurer, educational institution, or licensing body may justify a restriction by saying that it seeks to prevent risk. Sometimes there is a genuine reason to assess capacity or safety; the problem arises when diagnosis itself replaces individualized assessment. This is the same pattern already encountered in hospitalization: a medical category becomes a shortcut for evaluating a person.

One of the important principles of equality is therefore relevance. What information is truly required for the particular purpose? Does treatment years ago say anything about functioning today? Can the person be assessed on present functioning rather than diagnosis? Questions such as these reduce the possibility that psychiatry will follow someone like a permanent stamp long after their condition has changed.

Equality is also linked to the right not to be a hero. Public discourse often favors stories of 'overcoming,' in which a person with a mental disorder succeeds despite everything. Such stories can inspire hope, but they can also create an expectation that everyone must prove their worth through exceptional achievement. Genuine equality includes ordinary lives as well: an unremarkable job, a need for assistance, periods of reduced functioning, and gradual return. A person should not have to excel in order to be entitled to dignity and participation.

Equality is tested inside the health system as well. A person with a psychiatric history may come to a physician because of pain, shortness of breath, or another physical complaint, yet there is a risk that the mental-health information will affect how the complaint is interpreted. This phenomenon, sometimes called diagnostic overshadowing, occurs when a physical complaint is too quickly explained by the mental condition. This does not mean that mind-body connections are unreal; anxiety and depression can indeed influence physical symptoms. The problem begins when the psychiatric explanation closes the investigation instead of becoming one part of it.

Equality therefore means more than the right to enter the service. It also means the right to be taken seriously within it. The same principle works in the opposite direction: a medical system focused only on the body may overlook psychological distress because the person presented with another problem. Genuine integration requires the ability to see both layers without allowing one to cancel the other.

The same is true in encounters with public authorities. A person who struggles to complete a form or attend an appointment should not have to prove from the beginning every time that the difficulty is 'real.' A good accommodation mechanism reduces bureaucracy precisely where bureaucracy itself may be a barrier. Equality then becomes a matter of designing services in advance, not only correcting them after a discrimination complaint. An inclusive society does not wait for every person to fight alone for an adjustment; it builds frameworks on the assumption that people participate in different ways.

In this sense, the equality law changes the perspective of the book. Until this point, the discussion has focused mainly on the limits of state power and on rights during treatment. From here, a broader question enters: what is required for a person to live in the community as a citizen, rather than merely to be discharged from an institution? The answer leads directly to the rehabilitation revolution - to housing, employment, education, and relationships that give liberty practical substance.

Chapter Sixteen

The Community Rehabilitation Revolution

2000: A Change in Perspective

The Community Rehabilitation of Persons with Mental Disabilities Law, 5760-2000 - renamed by a 2024 amendment as the Community Rehabilitation of Persons Coping with Mental Health Conditions Law - was one of the major turning points in Israeli mental-health policy. The law was published on July 21, 2000 and entered into force on January 21, 2001.

Its purpose, as stated in the statute, is to advance rehabilitation and integration in the community so as to enable the greatest possible degree of functional independence and quality of life while preserving human dignity. The very language differs from the language of hospitalization laws. The focus is not dangerousness, authority, or an order of hospitalization; it is life.

What does a person need in order to live in the community? To work? To study? To build relationships? To manage a day? To receive support without being hospitalized? These are rehabilitation questions, and they change the standard by which the success of the system is measured.

The older model tended to measure success primarily through symptoms: has psychosis diminished, has mood improved, is the person taking medication? These measures matter, but they do not tell us whether the person has a home, work, friends, a sense of meaning, or control over life.

The rehabilitation law brings functioning and quality of life to the center. A person may continue to experience some symptoms and still live a full and meaningful life. Conversely, a person may be clinically stable while remaining isolated, unemployed, and entirely dependent on family.

This recognition lies at the foundation of the recovery model discussed later in the book: the system's purpose is not to return the person to one prescribed template of 'normality,' but to enable the person to build a life that they themselves regard as valuable.

The law created a framework for a basket of rehabilitation services. Areas of rehabilitation include, among other things, housing, employment, completion of education, social and leisure activities, support for families, care coordination, and additional services designed to support community integration.

The importance of the rehabilitation basket lies not only in the number of services. It expresses recognition that severe mental illness may affect many areas of life and that the response must therefore be multidimensional. Medication is not a substitute for housing; psychotherapy is not a substitute for work; hospitalization is not a substitute for community.

Housing is one of the most important foundations of recovery. A person who does not know where they will live after discharge finds it difficult to build a stable treatment plan. Supported-housing arrangements are intended to provide varying degrees of independence according to need.

Care is needed, however, to ensure that a rehabilitation service does not become a small institution in the community. If a housing framework manages almost every aspect of residents' lives, restricts choices unnecessarily, and conditions housing on complete compliance, it may reproduce institutional patterns outside hospital walls. The question is not only where the person lives, but how much control they have over life in that place.

Work and education are not only sources of income and knowledge. They provide identity, structure, belonging, and a sense of competence. For many years, people with severe mental disorders were effectively excluded from employment and educational settings on the assumption that the demands were too great for them.

Modern rehabilitation seeks to reverse the logic: rather than asking whether a person is 'ready' for life, it builds support that enables participation in life now. Supported employment, completion of education, and educational support reflect that approach.

In Israel, the family has an especially central role. Family members accompany people to treatment, monitor medication, provide a roof over their heads, and cope with crises. Family support can be an enormous resource, but it can also become a heavy burden if the state assumes that families will provide, without pay, what the service system does not.

The rehabilitation law also recognizes the need to support families. That recognition matters because rehabilitation does not occur in isolation, but also because autonomy should not depend on whether a person happens to have a strong and available family.

Eligibility and Its Limits

Like every social statute, the rehabilitation law defines conditions of eligibility. This creates a tension: on the one hand, a mechanism is needed to allocate resources; on the other, a person may need rehabilitation services even without meeting a particular formal threshold.

The tension points to a broader policy problem: treatment and rehabilitation are not always divided according to a person's actual needs, but according to boundaries between systems, budgets, and eligibility definitions. People who fall 'between the cracks' may receive too little treatment to prevent deterioration and too little rehabilitation to build a stable life.

In 2024, the Hebrew title of the law was changed from the equivalent of 'Community Rehabilitation of the Mentally Disabled' to language centered on persons coping with mental-health conditions. The change did not remake the entire system of rights, but language matters. The newer wording seeks to avoid a definition that makes disability or illness the person's central identity.

The change came almost a quarter of a century after the law was enacted, illustrating how social conceptions can change even within the statute book. Terms that were accepted in 2000 may, by 2024, be experienced as inconsistent with contemporary principles of dignity and equality.

The connection between rehabilitation and coercion is not always direct, but it is deep. The more community services exist, the more often a crisis can be identified early, continuous treatment can be provided, and deterioration ending in involuntary hospitalization can be prevented.

A policy aimed at reducing coercion therefore cannot focus only on amending sections of hospitalization law. If a person waits months for treatment, receives no support at home, and has no suitable housing arrangement, the hospital system will continue to function as the final safety net.

The rehabilitation law therefore pointed in a new direction: liberty is not protected only in the courtroom. It is also protected through services that enable a person to remain in the community.

The great innovation of the rehabilitation law was recognition that community rehabilitation warranted a statutory framework rather than being a form of charity dependent on local budgetary availability. This changes the relationship between the individual and the state. Housing, employment, and social participation are no longer merely 'ancillary services' provided after medical treatment has ended; they are recognized as part of the rehabilitation process itself.

Eligibility alone, however, does not guarantee fit. One person may need intensive housing support, another mainly employment assistance, and a third help with studies. Recovery-oriented rehabilitation should resist the temptation to construct a single pathway through which every person passes the same stations. The question is not which framework happens to be available, but what goal the person seeks and what minimum support will enable progress toward it.

Housing is one of the areas in which the difference between rehabilitation and control can be subtle. A housing framework can offer security, staff presence, and social connection; it can also create dependency and place everyday life under external rules.

The challenge is to create a continuum. Some people need, for a particular period, a setting with substantial staff presence; others can live independently with only occasional visits. Movement between levels of support should be possible in both directions, without a temporary deterioration erasing years of independence and without improvement forcing someone to leave a place they regard as home merely because the service is organized around fixed 'stages.'

Employment and education are more than instruments for improving income. They are sources of identity, belonging, and competence. For many years, rehabilitation systems tended to direct people toward sheltered employment or separate settings. More contemporary models seek, where this fits the person's wishes, to support participation in the ordinary labor market or mainstream educational settings.

This change is both legal and social. A person is not required to 'prove recovery' before being permitted to participate. Participation itself can be part of recovery.

Family can be the most important source of support, but it can also carry exhaustion, fear, and anger. A good rehabilitation service does not use the family as an inexpensive substitute for the system. It provides family members with knowledge, support, and space of their own while respecting the fact that an adult person does not belong to the family.

The balance is particularly complex in Israeli society, where family relationships often play a central role in care. Involvement can greatly improve continuity, but it must be built on a distinction between support and control, and between concern and the right to decide.

Rehabilitation as Protection Against Rehospitalization

From the perspective of this book, the rehabilitation law is also part of a policy against coercion. A person with stable housing, employment, connection to a team, and a meaningful routine may recognize deterioration earlier and receive help before a crisis reaches an extreme point.

Successful rehabilitation is often built from things that do not appear medical at all. A person begins getting up in the morning because work is waiting; adheres to treatment because they want to keep an independent apartment; learns to identify signs of crisis because there is a course of study they do not want to lose. Housing, employment, and education are therefore not rewards received after mental health improves. They can be part of the mechanism that enables improvement.

This approach also changes the balance of power. In a narrow medical model, professionals define clinical goals: fewer symptoms, fewer hospitalizations, greater adherence to treatment. In rehabilitation, the person is also asked to define personal goals: to become a present parent again, complete a course, live alone, build an intimate relationship, or simply use public transportation without fear. A goal may appear small from the outside but, for the person, it may be the most accurate measure that life is becoming their own again.

Even a rehabilitation service can become institutional if it rests on an expectation of compliance. When housing, work, or support is conditioned on behaving exactly as the system wants, the boundary between rehabilitation and supervision becomes blurred. Respectful rehabilitation requires tolerance for choices that are not always optimal, room for trial and error, and memory of the fact that the goal is not to create a 'good patient' but a citizen living their own life.

A major challenge is continuity. An achievement built over months can be damaged quickly if a framework closes, a staff member changes, or eligibility is lost. Rehabilitation should therefore not be a collection of temporary projects but a stable part of the health and welfare system. If the state seeks to reduce hospitalization, it must invest with equal seriousness in the life that takes place between hospitalizations.

Successful rehabilitation is often measured in moments that do not look 'therapeutic' at all: traveling alone by bus after a long period of difficulty, cooking again, persisting with a course, or meeting a friend once a week. For the individual, these may be more meaningful than a small shift on a clinical scale. A rehabilitation system that understands this begins with the life the person wants to build, not only with the deficits the system identifies.

This approach also requires patience with a non-linear pace. Rehabilitation is not a path in which every stage necessarily leads to greater independence. A person may progress at work while struggling with housing, need increased support after a crisis, and later return to a previous level of independence. A system that interprets every setback as failure may punish the person for needing help. A good continuum allows support to increase without erasing gains already made.

Here the deeper significance of rehabilitation in relation to coercion becomes clear. The more relationships, structure, and resources a person has, the more options exist before hospitalization. A friend who notices a change, a staff member who knows the early warning signs, stable housing, and a flexible employment setting can create time - and time is sometimes the difference between a crisis that can be managed by agreement and one that reaches an emergency. The rehabilitation basket is therefore not separate from the story of liberty; it is one of the foundations that allow liberty to survive periods of vulnerability.

Investment in rehabilitation is therefore not something that comes 'after' hospitalization; it is prevention of the next hospitalization. A system that assesses the cost of rehabilitation only by the number of service hours misses the potential benefit of fewer hospitalizations, preservation of functioning, and stronger independence.

Part Six

The Twenty-First Century: From Hospitalization to Recovery

Chapter Seventeen

Mental Health Reform in Israel

A Historical Separation Between Body and Mind

For many years, mental-health services in Israel were managed within a structure that was largely separate from general medicine. While the health funds played a central role in physical healthcare, a substantial share of responsibility for mental-health services remained with the state.

This separation reflected a historical tradition, but it carried costs. It reinforced the sense that mental health belonged to a different system, with different entry points and a separate stigma. In addition, when body and mind are treated in separate systems, continuity of care can suffer.

The National Health Insurance Law created a basis for discussing the transfer of responsibility as early as the 1990s, but implementation was delayed for many years. Only on July 1, 2015, was full insurance responsibility for inpatient and community mental-health services transferred to the health funds, apart from specific services that remained under the responsibility of the Ministry of Health.

Behind the reform lies an apparently simple principle: a mental disorder is a health condition, and therefore its treatment should be integrated into the general healthcare system. A patient should not have to become a citizen of a separate system merely because the affected organ cannot be seen on an X-ray.

Integration has the potential to reduce stigma, improve coordination between family medicine and psychiatry, and create clear responsibility on the part of the health fund toward its members. It can also make earlier identification of distress possible in a setting where the person is already receiving physical healthcare.

The transfer of legal and budgetary responsibility does not, by itself, guarantee availability. The test of the reform is what the patient encounters in practice: how long is the wait for a psychiatrist or psychotherapy? Is there a service in the area where the person lives? Is treatment suited to the person's language and culture? Is there continuity between hospitalization and community care?

Long waiting times are not merely a service problem. In mental health, they can become a rights problem. A condition that could have been treated at an early stage may worsen into a crisis. In this sense, access to voluntary treatment is directly connected to the prevention of coercion.

Mental-health services require skilled personnel. When psychiatrists, psychologists, social workers, and other therapists are concentrated in certain regions, the right to treatment is not realized equally.

A geographic gap is also a social gap. A person with financial means can sometimes turn to private care while waiting for a public service. Someone who cannot afford to pay must wait. In this way, a universal system can in practice create two speeds of treatment.

One of the central questions raised by the reform is who is responsible for a person as they move between settings. A psychiatric hospitalization may be brief, but if there is no timely appointment for follow-up care after discharge, the gains achieved during admission may erode.

Continuity of care requires more than a discharge letter. It requires communication between teams, an available appointment, orderly medication management, links with rehabilitation services, and a crisis plan. When every component is held by a different body, the person and their family may end up becoming the coordinators of the system themselves.

Integration into general medicine does not mean that mental health does not require unique expertise. A psychotic crisis, suicidality, or complex trauma is not the same as hypertension.

The goal is not to erase the distinctiveness of the field, but to end unnecessary institutional and social separation.

The challenge is to create a system in which mental-health treatment is a natural part of the health basket while still receiving the workforce, time, and settings appropriate to it.

The Reform from a Rights Perspective

Reforms are often measured in numbers: budgets, numbers of visits, and numbers of beds. From a rights perspective, additional questions must be asked: can the person choose? Is the service accessible? Does the person receive information? Is care provided in the community before hospitalization becomes necessary? Is there discrimination between those who can pay and those who cannot?

This is how the systemic discussion connects to autonomy. Freedom of choice is not real if the only option available in time is the emergency room. A system that seeks to reduce coercion must invest in accessible voluntary services long before the moment of crisis.

The transfer of responsibility to the health funds was intended, among other things, to break down the historical separation between body and mind. A person living with diabetes and depression is not two separate entities being treated by two separate systems; the health fund that knows the person's physical care should also be responsible for the mental-health pathway.

Integration has potential advantages: the family physician can identify distress early, refer to an appropriate service, and monitor the physical side effects of psychiatric treatment. A shared information system can improve continuity. Financing through the health basket also places mental health alongside other fields of medicine rather than treating it as a separate welfare budget.

But integration also creates questions of privacy. Psychiatric information is especially sensitive, and patients may fear broad disclosure within a medical system. The challenge is not to choose between continuity and privacy, but to create permissions, rules, and a culture of use that allow coordinated care without making a psychiatric diagnosis accessible to people who do not need it.

One measure of the success of reform is increased access: more people receive treatment. But an increase in the number of people entering the system is not enough. Waiting times, number of sessions, clinical fit, dropout, continuity, and disparities between populations must also be examined.

If more people enter the system but each person receives less time or waits longer, the increase alone does not prove that the service has improved. On the other hand, criticism based only on the number of sessions also requires caution: not every person needs long-term treatment. An efficient system should match the intensity of treatment to need rather than promise one uniform pathway.

Primary care has an important role in mental health. Common anxiety and depression often first appear in the family physician's office, and integrating mental-health professionals into primary-care clinics can reduce stigma and make access easier.

But an accessible gateway can also become a bottleneck if the family physician lacks time, training, or referral options. Integration therefore requires a direct connection between primary care and mental-health teams, rapid consultation, and clear urgent-care pathways.

On its face, the 2015 reform concerns insurance and community services rather than involuntary hospitalization. In practice, it is deeply connected to it. A health fund that succeeds in providing early care, monitoring, and continuity after discharge can reduce crises. A fund that struggles to provide a response pushes part of the burden toward emergency departments.

Responsibility for reducing coercion therefore does not belong only to the district psychiatrist or the hospital. It begins as well with decisions by the health funds about the geographic distribution of clinics, staffing, arrangements with providers, and alternatives to hospitalization.

2024 and Beyond: An Opportunity for Correction

The national program that began in 2024, accompanied by a substantial budget increase, was intended to expand the response during a period of exceptional demand. The development of crisis teams, home hospitalization, ACT, and crisis-respite houses points to an important shift: the community is no longer only the place to which people are discharged after hospitalization, but also a place where intensive care can be delivered during crisis.

For a person seeking care, the organizational structure is experienced through very simple questions: whom do I call, how long do I wait, how many times must I retell my story, and does the person I meet at the first appointment continue to accompany me later? A reform can be successful administratively and still feel cumbersome if the person must move from a call center to a family physician, to an initial assessment, to a clinic, and then to a new therapist at each stage.

Continuity does not mean that all treatment must be provided by the same professional. It means that the system should remember the story even when the patient moves between services. When responsibility changes hands, information, the treatment plan, and the person's preferences should move with it. Otherwise, precisely when someone is struggling to organize life, they are required to become their own case manager.

The transfer of responsibility to the health funds also changed the door through which a person enters the system. When mental health is more fully integrated into general medicine, a person can in principle turn to a family physician, receive a referral, and continue to treatment without entering a system perceived as a separate world. This integration has a stigma-reducing significance: anxiety or depression can be treated as part of the continuum of health rather than as an event that removes the person from “ordinary medicine.”

Organizational integration, however, does not guarantee integration in the lived experience. If the wait for a psychiatrist is long, if psychological treatment is limited, or if the person is repeatedly sent between providers, the system is still experienced as fragmented.

Mental-health care sometimes requires continuity that is difficult to achieve through isolated appointments. A crisis does not respect clinic hours, and deterioration can occur between visits. The quality of the system is therefore also measured by what happens in the intervals: who answers the phone, who notices when someone drops out, and who reaches out when a person stops attending.

The reform also raised questions of incentives. A system that finances services must decide how much to invest in short-term versus long-term treatment, community care versus hospitalization, and individual versus group treatment. These are not merely accounting decisions. They determine what kind of care will actually be available.

Transparency regarding waiting times, scope of service, and continuity of care is therefore part of the protection of rights, even if it is not usually framed in constitutional language.

Integration into general medicine can also change the first moment of seeking help. A person who notices worsening sleep, anxiety, or difficult thoughts may agree to discuss them with a family physician long before they would have approached a psychiatric clinic. If the physician knows how to identify warning signs, provide an initial response, and refer quickly when needed, treatment begins earlier and in a less threatening environment. In that sense, organizational reform can also influence culture: mental health becomes part of health, not a parallel system entered only when everything has already worsened.

The major advantage of the reform is the possibility of seeing the person as a whole. Mental and physical conditions affect one another, and psychiatric medications sometimes require physical monitoring. A system that connects these fields can improve care. The challenge is to ensure that integration does not turn mental health into just another service competing for time and resources within an already overloaded system.

The 2015 reform also changed the map of responsibility. Before responsibility was transferred to the health funds, it was easier to point to "the mental-health system" as a separate unit. After the reform, responsibility is distributed among primary care, mental-health clinics, providers, hospitals, and rehabilitation services. This dispersion has an advantage: mental health becomes part of general health. It also has a cost: when a person falls between frameworks, it becomes harder to know who is supposed to hold the continuity.

Continuity is the test through which organizational reforms become a personal experience. A person does not experience a "basket" or a "funding mechanism"; they experience whether there is an appointment, whether the next therapist knows their story, whether medications are recorded in the file, and whether someone calls after discharge. A system can improve in budgetary indicators and still leave a person feeling that they must coordinate between bodies that do not speak to one another.

This is especially important after a crisis. The first weeks after hospitalization require a delicate transition from an intensive setting back to ordinary life. If the community appointment is distant, if no provider knows the discharge plan, or if responsibility is handed to the family without support, the risk of a return to the emergency department rises. The question of reform is therefore not only who finances treatment, but who bears responsibility when a person moves between different levels of need.

A truly integrated system is one in which transitions between settings do not create breaks in continuity of care.

The success of this phase will be measured by the ability to turn programs into stable services. An emergency service must be known to the public, available outside regular hours, and connected to whoever continues the treatment after the crisis has passed.

Chapter Eighteen

The Recovery Model: The Person Beyond the Diagnosis

What Is "Recovery"?

In ordinary medical language, recovery may be understood as a return to the state that existed before illness or as the disappearance of symptoms. In mental health, however, a broader concept of Recovery has developed over recent decades. It does not promise that every symptom will disappear, nor does it make "complete cure" a condition for a good life.

Recovery in this sense is a personal process through which a person rebuilds control, hope, identity, relationships, and meaning. A person may continue to experience symptoms and still work, love, study, parent, create, and participate in the community.

The distinction may appear semantic, but it changes the purpose of treatment. Instead of asking only "How do we reduce the symptoms?" the question also becomes "What kind of life does this person want to build, and what can the system do to help?"

In a traditional medical model, goals are set mainly by professionals: stability, adherence to treatment, and prevention of hospitalization. These are important goals. But the person may see a different goal as central: returning to studies, rebuilding a relationship with their children, working, moving into an independent apartment, or reducing a side effect that interferes with daily life.

The recovery model does not eliminate medical expertise. It changes its place. The clinician is an expert in professional knowledge; the person is an expert in the experience of their own life and in what matters to them. A good treatment plan must connect these two forms of expertise.

Hope can sound too soft a concept for health policy, but in rehabilitation it has practical significance. If a team assumes that a person will never be able to work or live independently, that assumption will influence the opportunities offered. If the person internalizes it, the assumption may become self-fulfilling.

Hope is not a promise and does not ignore difficulty. It is the recognition that a diagnosis does not predetermine the limits of the life that remains possible.

Hospitalization and diagnosis can reduce a person to the role of "patient." A medical record mainly documents problems: symptoms, risks, medications, and admissions. It does not necessarily record that the person is also a teacher, a parent, a musician, a friend, or someone with dreams.

The recovery model seeks to restore that broader identity. This also matters therapeutically: meaningful goals may motivate change more powerfully than a general demand to "remain stable."

One development associated with the recovery model is the inclusion of people with personal lived experience of mental-health difficulties within treatment and rehabilitation services. A peer specialist is not merely an "inspirational story." Such a person can bring knowledge that the professional system cannot acquire from textbooks: how hospitalization is experienced, how a conversation with staff feels during crisis, what helps build trust, and what is experienced as humiliating.

The inclusion of peers also changes the structure of authority. It brings into the system a voice that does not come only from the treating side.

A genuine tension appears here. The recovery model emphasizes choice, self-direction, and partnership; involuntary hospitalization rests on the possibility that the state may replace a person's choice with its own decision. The contradiction cannot be resolved by a slogan.

Even a system that accepts the possibility of coercion in extreme situations can be recovery-oriented if it minimizes coercion as much as possible, explains the decision, preserves choice in areas where choice remains possible, and begins planning the return of control to the person already during the crisis.

By contrast, a system that uses the language of "recovery" while continuing to make decisions without the person has not truly changed the balance of power. Recovery is not a poster on the wall; it is a test of how the service actually operates.

Recovery Is Not Linear

A person may make progress and later experience another crisis. A repeated hospitalization does not necessarily mean that all previous progress has been erased. A linear view of success and failure can create shame and reduce willingness to try again.

Recovery is often a process of adaptation: the person learns to identify early warning signs, understand what helps, decide who should be present during a crisis, and build a plan that reduces harm.

This leads directly to the next idea: if we recognize the person as an expert in their own life when they are stable, can we respect their preferences as well if they later enter a crisis? Supported decision-making and advance directives attempt to answer that question.

One reason the term "Recovery" initially caused confusion is that in medical language "recovery" sounds like the disappearance of illness. In the recovery model, the meaning is broader. A person may continue to experience symptoms, need medication, or require support, and still build a life they regard as worthwhile.

This emphasis changes the purpose of the service. If the only goal is symptom reduction, a team may prefer stability even at the price of fatigue, dependence, or abandonment of personal goals. If the goal includes meaningful life, the system must explore with the person what price they are willing to pay for stability and what they most want to preserve.

None of this minimizes symptoms. Psychosis, depression, and anxiety can be severe and disabling. The recovery model simply refuses to give them exclusive authority over the definition of success.

“Hope” can sound like a soft concept that does not belong in policy. In practice, the expectations of professionals influence the opportunities they offer. If a team assumes that a person with a particular diagnosis will never be able to work, study, or live independently, it may direct them toward restricted settings before the person has even had the opportunity to try.

A recovery-oriented approach does not guarantee any particular outcome, but it keeps possibilities open. It replaces a prophecy of limitation with ongoing assessment of risk, support, and progress.

Including people with lived experience in mental-health services gently challenges the traditional hierarchy of knowledge. The physician holds medical knowledge; the social worker holds systemic knowledge; the psychologist holds therapeutic knowledge; and the peer holds another kind of knowledge - what it feels like to be the person receiving a diagnosis, what a locked ward feels like, and what helps a person return to life after crisis.

This knowledge does not replace research or professional training. It complements them. When a team designs a service without the presence of people who have experienced it, it is easy to miss details that appear small from the outside but are decisive from within: the tone in which information is given, access to a telephone, the degree of privacy, or the way a search of belongings is carried out.

Treatment systems naturally tend to minimize risk. But a life without risk is impossible, and overprotection can itself obstruct development. A person who wants to return to work, live alone, or manage their own money may fail. The question is whether every risk justifies prevention.

The recovery model speaks of positive risk-taking - accepting calculated risk as part of building independence. This does not mean ignoring serious danger, but recognizing that autonomy includes the possibility of making mistakes and trying again.

Here rehabilitation and rights meet. A system that prevents every person with a history of crisis from making choices that involve some degree of risk may preserve dependence precisely in the name of protection.

Outcome Measures from the Person's Perspective

To implement the model, measurement must also change. The rate of readmission is an important measure, but it is not enough. A person who has not been hospitalized again because they never leave home is not necessarily a "success." Quality of life, relationships, employment, sense of control, belonging, and the ability to pursue personal goals must also be considered.

The recovery model emerged in large part from the gap between what a system can measure and what a person experiences. Clinically, a record may show fewer symptoms, fewer hospitalization days, and improved functioning. Yet the person may say that life still feels empty, that meaningful relationships are absent, and that the entire daily routine is organized around mental-health services.

Conversely, a person who still hears voices or experiences fluctuations in mood may learn to live with them, work, build relationships, and feel that life has meaning. Both pictures can be true at the same time.

Recovery, then, is not a softer version of "positive thinking." It does not impose a moral duty on the person to feel well, nor does it suggest that everyone can recover if they only want it enough. Mental-health conditions may be severe, chronic, and limiting. Medication, therapy, and professional services remain important. The innovation is that the system is not entitled to define success solely from its own perspective. The person also has authority to say what counts, for them, as a good life.

There is also a danger that recovery itself will become an institutional slogan. If a service requires a person to present "recovery goals" in fixed language, or measures them by how quickly they become independent, a liberating idea may be converted into a new demand. Sometimes recovery means progress; sometimes it means maintaining stability; and sometimes it means getting through a difficult period without losing one's home, relationships, or dignity.

One of the challenges of the recovery model is its relationship to risk. Medical systems naturally try to avoid failure, while independent life includes risk: trying a new job, moving home, entering a relationship, or reducing support. If every risk is interpreted as evidence that the person is "not ready," rehabilitation stops at precisely the point where it is supposed to become life.

Recovery therefore requires the system to distinguish between unreasonable danger and the ordinary risk every person takes when building a future.

The deeper meaning of the model is a change in identity. The person is not a project of the system. Professionals can accompany, advise, and assist, but the life toward which the process is directed is not theirs. Once this premise is accepted, the clinical question changes too: not only "Which treatment reduces symptoms?" but "What will help this person regain roles, relationships, choice, and a future?"

The recovery model also changes the relationship to time. Medicine tends to think in treatment episodes: hospitalization, a course of sessions, a medication change. Life is not divided that way. A person may feel that they are progressing for months and then experience a setback; return to work and discover that social difficulty remains; reduce symptoms yet still fear the next crisis. Recovery in the personal sense is not a straight line, but the ability to build continuity even when interruptions occur along the way.

One of the deepest changes is the possibility of holding an identity that is not ruled by the diagnosis. Early in the process, a person may explain every emotion through illness or fear that every excitement is a sign of deterioration. Later, they may learn to distinguish between different parts of themselves: they have a psychiatric history, but they are also a partner, a worker, a football fan, a parent, or simply someone who wants peace and quiet. A good service does not erase the diagnosis; it returns it to dimensions proportionate to the rest of life.

Measures of recovery should therefore include a sense of control. Two people may have the same level of symptoms, yet one may feel that life is managed by the system while the other feels that they use services as tools. That difference is difficult to measure, but it matters. It explains why partnership in decisions is not merely an ethical value but part of recovery itself: the person relearns that they can influence the direction in which life moves.

Personal measures do not replace clinical data. They add the outcome for whose sake the clinical data mattered in the first place.

Chapter Nineteen

Supported Decision-Making: Assistance Instead of Substitution

From "Who Will Decide for Them?" to "What Will Help Them Decide?"

For many years, when a person had difficulty making significant decisions, the conventional legal response was the appointment of a guardian. The idea was protective: someone else would act in the person's best interests. But the cost was substantial - authority was transferred from the person to another decision-maker.

Amendment No. 18 to Israel's Legal Capacity and Guardianship Law, published in April 2016, marked a conceptual change. It strengthened alternatives to guardianship, including enduring powers of attorney and supported decision-making, and placed the person's will, independence, and autonomy at the center.

Supported decision-making rests on a simple idea: difficulty understanding or deciding is not necessarily a reason to replace the person. Sometimes the person needs information adapted to their needs, an explanation, time, a trusted person who can help compare alternatives, or practical help implementing the decision.

Under a supported decision-making arrangement, the person remains the decision-maker. The supporter may help gather information, understand it, weigh options, and carry out the choice, but is not supposed to replace the person's will with the supporter's own.

This distinction is fundamental. Support is not guardianship under a different name. If the supporter effectively decides what is "right" for the person, the model loses its defining feature.

The principle is especially relevant to mental health because decision-making capacity can fluctuate over time. A person may experience a period of crisis and later return to a high level of functioning. A flexible model of support is more compatible with that reality than a fixed model of substituted authority.

People make decisions with help from others all the time. They consult partners, friends, physicians, lawyers, and accountants. Needing assistance does not in itself negate independence.

The problem is that when a psychiatric diagnosis exists, ordinary human dependence can be interpreted differently. A need for explanation becomes “incapacity”; hesitation becomes “lack of insight.” A supported approach asks first what accommodations might enable the person to decide.

For example, a person in acute distress may understand information better in a short conversation and plain language than in a long legal document. They may need a break, a familiar person, or repeated explanation. Such accommodations do not manufacture capacity; they allow existing capacity to be expressed.

One of the most promising ideas in mental health is advance crisis planning. During a stable period, a person can describe what helped in the past, which medications caused severe side effects, whom they want contacted, what helps them calm down, which interventions they wish to avoid, and what their preferences are if they later have difficulty expressing them in real time.

Psychiatric advance directives exist in different forms around the world. Even where their legal force is not absolute, they offer an important ethical change: instead of treating the person’s wishes during crisis as irrelevant, the system tries to preserve wishes expressed when the person was able to articulate them clearly.

Such planning can also reduce conflict. A team that knows the person’s preferences in advance may be able to act in a way that produces less fear and less resistance.

The traditional model of guardianship relied heavily on the idea of the person's "best interests." The newer rights-based model places greater emphasis on the person's will and preferences. The difference is not theoretical.

A person's "best interests" can be defined by someone else according to values that are not the person's own. One person may prefer maximum stability even at the cost of side effects; another may prefer to accept a degree of risk in order to preserve alertness, creativity, or the ability to work. There is not always one medical answer to the question of what balance is right.

Respecting the person's will is therefore not an obstacle to treatment; it is part of defining what good treatment means.

The supported model also has limits. There are emergencies in which a lengthy process cannot be awaited; there are periods in which some people have great difficulty expressing a consistent preference; and there is a risk of pressure or exploitation by the supporter.

The answer is not to return automatically to substituted decision-making, but to build safeguards: choosing an appropriate supporter, supervision where needed, the ability to replace the supporter, and a clear distinction between assistance and improper influence.

Supported Decision-Making as a Challenge to Coercive Psychiatry

The idea of support poses a direct question to mental-health law: before the state decides against a person's wishes, has it done enough to enable the person to decide for themselves?

That question can change the order of actions. Instead of diagnosis -> refusal -> coercion, one can imagine a different pathway: distress -> clarification of the person's wishes -> adaptation of information -> support -> a less restrictive alternative -> and only if these are insufficient and the risk meets the legal threshold, consideration of coercion.

In this way, an amendment born in the law of legal capacity and guardianship reaches the heart of the mental-health debate. It does not repeal the Treatment of Mental Patients Law, but it offers a different conception of the person in situations of vulnerability: not someone whose will should quickly be replaced, but someone for whom a genuine effort should be made to remain the person making decisions about their own life.

The difference between guardianship and supported decision-making is first and foremost a difference in ownership of the decision. Under guardianship, to the extent the guardian is authorized, another person may make decisions on the individual's behalf. Under support, the person decides; the supporter assists in understanding information, weighing alternatives, communicating with institutions, and implementing the choice.

The distinction is practical, not theoretical. A supporter who disagrees with the decision is not supposed simply to replace it. The supporter's role is to help the person reach their own decision, to the extent possible within the law.

Support can be cognitive - breaking complex information into manageable parts; emotional - creating conditions in which the person can think without pressure; communicative - helping the person express their wishes; and practical - assisting in contact with a bank, physician, or public authority.

Timing is especially important in mental health. Decision-making capacity can change. A person who has great difficulty during a crisis may return within days or weeks to full capacity. A permanent legal solution may therefore be disproportionate to a temporary problem.

Even a mechanism designed to strengthen autonomy can become a form of control if the supporter is too dominant. A family member may say they are "helping" while actually steering the person toward the choice most convenient for the family. A professional can frame options so that only one appears reasonable.

Supported decision-making therefore requires ethical rules, oversight, and the person's ability to change supporters. Support must remain faithful to the person's will and preferences, not to the wishes of the person providing assistance.

The difficult question is what happens when the crisis itself profoundly impairs capacity. Support may then be insufficient. Even so, it can reduce the scope in which others need to decide.

A person may be unable at that moment to decide whether to leave a hospital, but still be able to choose who should be with them, which of two medications they prefer, when to speak with family, and what helps them calm down. Recognizing partial capacity prevents loss of authority in one area from spreading to every area of life.

An advance directive is, in a sense, a message from the person in a stable period to the person in crisis and to the team that will meet them. It allows the person to "support themselves" in advance by defining values, accumulated experience, and the things they want others to remember when speaking becomes difficult.

There is therefore a deep connection between supported decision-making and crisis planning. Both seek to extend the reach of autonomy beyond the moment in which capacity is full and obvious.

A Cultural Change Deeper Than Law

Recognition of support requires professionals to become comfortable with the fact that a good decision is not always the decision they themselves would make. This is a shift from a model in which the expert supplies the answer to one in which expertise serves the person in choosing the answer.

Supported decision-making can be understood through an everyday situation. A person experiencing severe depression must decide whether to move home, begin a new treatment, or return to work. They struggle to concentrate, feel overwhelmed by the options, and say to a sister, "Decide for me." A traditional model may see this as a sign that another person should receive authority. A supported model first asks what might help the person decide: break the decision into stages, write down the options, hold the conversation at a time of day when concentration is better, and ask the sister to assist without choosing in the person's place.

The difference may appear small, but it is profound. When another person makes the decision, the responsibility and outcome can feel foreign. When the person makes the decision with support, even extensive support, it remains part of the person's own life story. This is especially important in mental health, where a sense of control may already be damaged during crisis.

Over time, many families develop an "expertise of relatives." They learn to notice changes in tone of voice, sleeping patterns, unusual spending, or withdrawal that may precede deterioration. This knowledge can be extremely valuable, but it is not identical to the person's knowledge of themselves. A good system must know how to receive information from family without turning the family into the only spokesperson, and how to listen to the person without dismissing what relatives can see.

The balance is particularly complex when relationships themselves are strained. Not every family is a safe space, and not every relative who approaches the system necessarily represents the person's wishes. Supported decision-making therefore cannot rely on a formula of "involve the family"; it must ask whom the person chooses to involve, in what role, and within what limits.

Families often occupy the most difficult position. They have known the person for years, have seen previous deteriorations, and know what happened when treatment was refused. It is natural that they want influence. But family knowledge is not the same as the right to decide. Good support sometimes requires relatives to do something difficult: state clearly what they believe, warn about risk, and still leave room for the person to choose differently as long as the person is able to do so.

In extreme situations, supported decision-making does not solve every problem. When capacity is profoundly impaired and immediate risk exists, the law may permit intervention. But precisely because that possibility exists, it is important to build support before crisis: advance directives, a trusted person, preferences regarding treatment, and preferred places to seek help. In this way, part of autonomy can be preserved even when the ability to express it in real time is reduced.

Supported decision-making becomes clearer when we stop imagining a decision as a single isolated moment. In life, people almost never decide entirely alone. They ask family members, consult professionals, read information, and ask for time. Independence is not isolation. The key question is who ultimately holds authority over the choice, and when it is permissible to transfer that authority to someone else.

In a mental-health crisis, prior familiarity has special value. A supporter who knows the person during stable periods may know that they need quiet before a conversation, that physical contact increases distress, or that a particular medication previously caused severe side effects. This knowledge does not give the supporter the right to decide in the person's place, but it can help the team interpret behavior and find a way to communicate. Support thus becomes not only a legal tool but a bridge between the person in ordinary life and the person during crisis.

The challenge is to avoid turning support into a route that bypasses autonomy. The closer the supporter is, the more they may also carry fears and interests of their own. A family member may seek a solution that protects the household even when the person would prefer something else. Good support therefore requires separating "what I think is best" from "what this person wants and what will help them understand." That separation is not always easy, but it is the heart of the model: helping the person remain the decision-maker, not merely receiving a decision written for them in gentler language.

None of this removes professional responsibility. A physician must still recommend, warn, and act in emergencies according to law. But the starting point changes: disagreement is not a malfunction that needs to be corrected. It is a possible part of an encounter between two people who hold different forms of knowledge and different roles.

Part Seven

Coercion Under the Test of Human Rights

Chapter Twenty

Involuntary Hospitalization in the Twenty-First Century

The Exception That Defines the Limits of the System

Involuntary psychiatric hospitalization is one of the places where the power of the state is felt most directly in a person's body. A person may be taken from where they are, examined against their wishes, and kept in a ward they are not free to leave. It is not necessary to minimize the seriousness of that act in order to recognize that it is sometimes intended to prevent catastrophe.

The challenge for a modern system is not to choose between two slogans - "never coerce" or "protect at any cost" - but to define strict conditions, act only for the shortest period required, and repeatedly examine whether the infringement remains justified.

In Israel, the authority for involuntary hospitalization may arise, depending on the circumstances, from the district psychiatrist, the director of a psychiatric institution in limited circumstances, or a court. Each route rests on a different legal source of authority and different mechanisms of review.

The basic principle should be clear: a person must not be hospitalized involuntarily merely because they have a psychiatric diagnosis. A diagnosis may be relevant to understanding the person's condition, but it is not by itself proof of dangerousness, impaired judgment, or a need to deprive the person of liberty.

Under the relevant Israeli compulsory-treatment pathways, the law requires a connection between the mental condition and a significant impairment in judgment or reality testing, together with additional conditions involving danger or serious harm.

The Ministry of Health explains the process to the public in terms of psychotic states, dangerousness or suicidality, and refusal of voluntary hospitalization; the precise legal wording is found in the statute itself.

The distinction between a public explanation and the wording of the law matters. Rights cannot rest on a pedagogical shorthand. When liberty is being deprived, the precise statutory conditions govern.

Dangerousness is a central concept in hospitalization law. There is no doubt that behavior, thoughts, planning, clinical history, and surrounding circumstances can sometimes create a genuine risk. But risk assessment is probabilistic, not prophetic.

Error can operate in both directions. Underestimating risk may lead to harm that could have been prevented. Overestimating risk may result in the loss of liberty of a person who would not have harmed themselves or others. When a system fears mainly the first type of error, it may develop a tendency to hospitalize "just to be safe." From a rights perspective, however, unnecessary hospitalization is also a real harm.

A proper risk assessment should therefore be individualized, current, and reasoned. It must distinguish between generalized dangerousness attributed to a group and the concrete risk posed by a particular person at a particular time.

The law distinguishes between urgent and non-urgent situations. When an immediate danger exists, the state may need to act quickly. There may be less time for explanation, an additional assessment, or coordination of community services.

Urgency, however, does not cancel dignity. Even when immediate action is required, it is still possible to explain what is being done, avoid force beyond what is necessary, allow contact with a person chosen by the individual where possible, and document the decision.

Precisely in the moments when the state exercises its greatest power, the highest human standard is required.

According to current Ministry of Health information, an involuntary hospitalization order issued by a district psychiatrist is initially given for up to seven days. An extension of a further seven days may be sought, and continued hospitalization beyond fourteen days requires referral to the district psychiatric committee.

These numbers are not merely procedural. They express a principle: the longer the infringement continues, the more it requires a renewed and more independent justification.

A hospitalization that was justified on the first day may become unjustified on the tenth if the risk has passed and an appropriate alternative exists.

The person's ability and willingness to engage with treatment may also change. Someone who arrived agitated and confused may, after several days, be able to converse, understand, and choose. The status of "involuntarily hospitalized patient" must not become a fixed identity for the entire admission.

An order of the district psychiatrist may be appealed to the district psychiatric committee, and decisions of the committee are subject to judicial review in the district court in accordance with the law. The right to state-funded legal representation strengthens the possibility that the process will not be one-sided.

Effective review should examine not only whether the person is "ill," but the entire chain of justification: are the statutory conditions met? What is the risk? On what facts is it based? Is there a connection to the mental condition? What has changed since the previous decision? What alternatives exist?

The Least Restrictive Alternative

The principle of proportionality requires thinking in steps. If the person can be protected through intensive home treatment, a crisis-respite house, safe family support, a crisis clinic, or an open setting, those options should be considered seriously before using a locked ward.

The difficulty is that a legal alternative exists only when a therapeutic alternative exists in reality. A committee cannot meaningfully be asked to release a person to "the community" when there is no appointment, no framework, and no provider ready to receive them. The protection of liberty is therefore directly connected to budgetary policy.

Even a hospitalization that saved a life can be experienced as traumatic. A person may remember the transport, the locked door, the use of force, or the feeling that no one believed them. If the system ignores the experience because it believes the decision was correct, it may damage the trust required for future treatment.

After a crisis, there is value in discussing what happened: what led to the hospitalization, what helped, what caused harm, and what might be done differently next time. Such a conversation is not an admission that the hospitalization was unjustified. It is recognition that even a justified intervention may carry a cost.

The division between voluntary and involuntary hospitalization appears clear in legal documents, but in practice there are intermediate situations. A person may agree to admission after being told that, if they refuse, an involuntary order may be considered. Sometimes this is a legitimate explanation of the legal situation; at other times it creates a form of “consent” in which no real alternative exists.

From a rights perspective, staff must distinguish persuasion from threat. If a genuine legal basis for coercion exists, it can be explained. But the possibility of coercion should not be used routinely to obtain a signature.

Meaningful consent requires that the person understand their status, what will happen if they ask to leave, and what rights they have.

The Israeli framework uses time-limited stages and therefore recognizes the principle that the justification for hospitalization must be re-examined. The importance of time limits is not merely procedural. A psychiatric condition can change rapidly. A person who arrived in severe turmoil may stabilize within days, and a justification that was strong on the first night may weaken.

Every extension should therefore be examined as though it were a new decision, not as an automatic continuation. The question is not "Was it justified to hospitalize?" but "Is it justified to keep this person hospitalized today?"

Involuntary hospitalization removes freedom to leave, but it does not remove every other right. A person does not automatically lose the rights to privacy, contact with loved ones, information, everyday choices, and participation in treatment.

It is important to distinguish between restrictions imposed for safety and restrictions that arise only from organizational convenience. Even on a locked ward, there can be choice regarding activity times, food, clothing, telephone contact, and treatment preferences unless there is an individualized reason to restrict them.

This preserves an important principle: coercion in one domain must not "spread" across the whole of a person's life.

Coercive decisions often depend on predictions about the future. Yet no tool can predict with certainty who will harm themselves or others. When the perceived cost of error is catastrophe, a system will naturally prefer to "err on the side of safety." But that approach has a cost: many people may lose their liberty in order to prevent an event that would never have occurred.

There is no complete mathematical solution. Protection lies in the combination of professional risk assessment, documentation, alternatives, limited duration, and review. The less certain the prediction, the more important it is that the intervention be reversible and short.

The Experience of Hospitalization Affects Future Treatment

A person who experiences involuntary hospitalization as humiliating may avoid seeking help early in the future, fearing that any disclosure of suicidal or psychotic thoughts will lead to admission. An action intended to protect in the short term can therefore increase risk over the longer term.

The ward itself can influence how the crisis develops. A noisy, crowded environment with little privacy can increase suspiciousness and arousal; a team that succeeds in creating predictability and personal connection can reduce them. Hospital conditions are therefore not merely a matter of comfort. They are part of the therapeutic environment and may influence the need for restrictive measures. Investment in space, staffing, and time for conversation is, in this sense, also an investment in reducing coercion.

The experience of involuntary hospitalization is shaped not only by the decision itself but also by the way it is carried out. The same order can produce two very different experiences. In one case, the person receives an explanation, is allowed to take essential belongings, a chosen relative is contacted, and staff speak respectfully. In another, the person receives short commands, does not understand where they are being taken, and experiences the event as an arrest. Legally the authority may be identical; humanly the difference is enormous.

Time is a central element of the decision. The justification for involuntary hospitalization should not become a label that continues by itself. Mental condition changes, sometimes quickly. A person who was highly agitated at night may be able to have a very different conversation in the morning. Periodic review is therefore not technical; it expresses the idea that a deprivation of liberty must be examined for as long as it continues. As the condition improves, the burden of justification must return to the system.

There is also a difference between “this person cannot be discharged” and “there is nowhere to discharge this person to.” If someone remains hospitalized because no housing framework, home treatment, or family support exists, a social problem effectively becomes a medical restriction of liberty. In such cases, investment in community services is not merely welfare policy; it is a means of reducing coercion. The choice between hospitalization and discharge becomes real only when a third option is available in time.

The quality of a coercive system is therefore measured as well by the number of cases that never reach coercion. A statute may regulate involuntary hospitalization well, but a better system is one that identifies deterioration early, intervenes gently, and builds trust so that a person agrees to receive help before the risk becomes extreme. In that sense, the test of involuntary hospitalization begins long before the hospitalization order.

Involuntary hospitalization often begins long before entry into the ward. A telephone call by a family member, a clinic visit, an ambulance request, or an encounter with police can all be links in the chain. Each link adds information, but each can also increase fear. When coordination is absent, the person retells the story to different people and every encounter starts from zero. A system that seeks to reduce coercion must view the route to hospitalization as part of the intervention.

The moment of transport is especially important. There is a difference between explaining where the person is going, allowing them to take a telephone and documents and contact someone they choose, and transferring them quickly without any understanding of what will happen. Sometimes risk leaves little room for flexibility, but even then small details of dignity can be preserved. They do not change the fact that the person does not consent; they change the degree of humiliation that accompanies the coercion.

Discharge is also part of involuntary hospitalization. If a person leaves the ward without understanding what led to the crisis, who will meet them next, and when, coercion ends legally but the system has not necessarily restored control. Good discharge planning seeks to turn the event into information: which warning signs appeared earlier, what helped, what was difficult, and whom to contact next time. In that way, hospitalization need not remain a closed chapter of "what was done to me," but can become - insofar as the person is ready - part of a plan that increases the chance that the next crisis will be managed earlier and with less force.

This is why a debriefing conversation after a coercive event matters: explaining what happened, hearing how the person experienced it, identifying what could have been done differently, and building a plan for the next crisis. Even when the harm cannot be undone, the event can be turned into a source of learning rather than an unprocessed rupture.

Chapter Twenty-One

Treatment Without Consent

Bodily Liberty Within a Loss of Freedom of Movement

The fact that a person is involuntarily hospitalized does not automatically answer a separate question: which treatments may be given without consent? Hospitalization and treatment are two distinct circles of intervention. The first removes the freedom to leave; the second acts directly upon the body and mind.

This distinction matters because there is an intuitive tendency to assume that once the state has decided that a person cannot decide whether to remain in hospital, it may also decide every treatment question on that person's behalf. A rights-based approach rejects that automatic expansion.

Even during involuntary hospitalization, the person should continue to be involved in the treatment plan, alternatives should be explained, and consent should be sought wherever possible. Coercive treatment must rest on legal authority and appropriate conditions, not merely on institutional convenience.

Psychiatric medication can reduce psychosis, anxiety, depression, agitation, and other symptoms. It can also cause side effects, and the person may experience the cost of those effects differently from the way the treatment team evaluates them.

When a patient refuses, the professional question is not merely how to make the person take the medication. It is necessary to understand why the person refuses. They may fear a side effect experienced in the past; they may not believe that they are ill; the medication may produce a sense of emotional blunting; or the refusal itself may arise from a psychotic belief.

Different reasons require different responses. A different medication, another dose, further explanation, more time, or a different route of administration can sometimes turn confrontation into agreement. Resorting to coercion too early may save time in the short term while imposing a cost in trust over the long term.

A patient on a locked ward exists within an asymmetrical relationship of power. The patient knows that staff hold authority regarding leave, conditions of hospitalization, and sometimes discharge. Even a “yes” to treatment must therefore be understood within that context.

Did the person understand that options existed? Was unnecessary pressure applied? Were side effects explained? Was there an opportunity to ask questions? Meaningful consent is not created merely because there was no physical resistance.

Electroconvulsive therapy (ECT) is a useful example of the gap between historical imagery and modern treatment. Historically, the treatment was given under conditions very different from those accepted today. Modern ECT is administered under anesthesia and with muscle relaxation, and there is evidence for its efficacy in some severe clinical conditions.

In Israel, the regulations under the Treatment of Mental Patients Law establish special conditions for ECT, including a decision by several physicians, a physical examination, and documentation of the reasons. The regulations require written consent when the patient is voluntarily hospitalized; treatment of an involuntarily hospitalized patient is governed by the special legal framework and has also been addressed in case law.

A rights-based discussion should not become a simplistic debate over whether ECT is “good” or “bad.” It is possible to recognize medical benefit while also requiring a high threshold of justification, explanation, and oversight when treatment is given against a person’s wishes.

In extreme emergencies there may be no time for a full consent process. Medicine generally recognizes situations in which urgent treatment is given to prevent serious harm. But "emergency" should describe a condition, not a culture of work.

If every difficulty on the ward is defined as an emergency, the exception becomes the rule. Documentation, retrospective review, and the question whether escalation could have been prevented through earlier intervention are therefore important.

Autonomy is not the right to choose only what the physician recommends. In ordinary life, people are permitted to make decisions that involve risk. They may refuse surgery, continue a harmful habit, or choose a less effective treatment, as long as the law recognizes their capacity to decide and they understand the implications.

Psychiatry should not become a domain in which every personal risk immediately justifies substituting another person's will. The threshold for intervention must remain tied to the legal conditions and to a genuine impairment in decision-making capacity or a level of risk that justifies the exception.

Consent Is Not a One-Time Event

Treatment that begins with consent still requires continuing consent. A patient may ask questions, request a change in dose, report side effects, and change their mind. A signed form is not an unlimited license to continue treatment.

This is especially important in psychiatry because treatment can affect alertness, energy, appetite, sexual functioning, and movement. From the patient's perspective, side effects may matter more than the improvement in symptoms that staff observe. A conversation about treatment should therefore ask not only "Is it working?" but also "What price are you paying for the effect?"

Autonomy is not exhausted by the right to refuse. Resistance can sometimes be reduced by offering genuine choice: another medication, a different dose, a different route of administration, complementary psychological treatment, or more time for discussion.

Even when the law permits treatment without consent, a space for choice should be preserved within the framework. If two medications are appropriate, the patient's preference regarding side effects should carry weight. This helps preserve a sense of control even where the larger decision has been restricted.

There is a moral and legal difference between an immediate act intended to save life and continuing treatment intended to improve a condition over time. In an emergency, when a person cannot express consent and immediate danger exists, time itself restricts the possibility of discussion. As treatment continues, the justification for relying on emergency alone becomes weaker.

A rights-based mechanism should therefore require increasing review when coerced treatment shifts from a brief intervention to an ongoing policy. The question "What did we do to prevent disaster tonight?" is not the same as "What treatment will be given over the coming weeks?"

One possible error in coerced treatment is to evaluate side effects only according to medical criteria. For a person whose work depends on fine motor control, a mild tremor may be highly significant; for another, weight gain may affect body image and physical health; a third person may prefer drowsiness to anxiety.

Even when treatment is given against the person's wishes, there remains a duty to continue asking what the person wants. The fact that the person did not make the final decision about whether treatment would be given does not mean that they have nothing to say about how it is provided.

The Dual Test

Treatment without consent must satisfy two separate tests: is it medically justified, and is the infringement of autonomy legally and ethically justified? A treatment may be effective yet unjustified if imposed; conversely, a situation may justify some form of intervention without justifying the particular treatment selected.

Refusal of treatment is not, by itself, proof of incapacity. A person may fully understand that medication could reduce symptoms and nevertheless fear weight gain, fatigue, sexual dysfunction, or a recurrence of side effects experienced previously. From the team's perspective, the cost may appear small compared with the risk of deterioration; from the person's perspective, it may be central. Informed consent requires taking seriously values that are not purely clinical.

This has particular significance in psychiatry because treatment can affect a person's sense of self. A person may say that a medication "flattens" them, makes them feel less creative, or leaves them feeling unlike themselves. Such experiences are difficult to quantify, but that does not make them irrelevant. Medicine that seeks partnership must be able to discuss not only efficacy but also the subjective price of treatment.

Sometimes resistance can be reduced through genuine choice: a different dose, another medication, a more gradual pace, psychotherapy alongside medication, or agreement on a trial period. In other cases, the disagreement remains.

Even then, there is value in ensuring that the person knows what has been decided, why, for how long, and how the decision can be reviewed. Treatment given under compulsion need not turn the entire encounter into a coercive relationship.

There is also value in acknowledging uncertainty. Patients sometimes hear absolute statements precisely where medicine itself operates in probabilities. A statement such as "This is my recommendation, but I cannot guarantee how you will respond" does not weaken professional authority; it can strengthen trust because it distinguishes knowledge from false certainty.

In a field where many people have experienced decisions being made for them, transparency about the limits of knowledge is part of partnership.

Trust damaged by treatment without consent is difficult to rebuild, but not necessarily lost. Once the person's condition stabilizes, a conversation can explore what the person remembers, what felt intolerable, and what might have been done differently. Sometimes it becomes clear that the objection was not to the treatment itself but to the way it was proposed. That knowledge can become a resource for the next crisis. Again, the boundary between ethics and treatment is not sharp: respectful conduct can also reduce the need for force in the future.

Refusal of treatment is sometimes a conversation about trust more than pharmacology. A person who refuses medication may be responding to a previous experience in which side effects were not heard, to fear that agreeing once will mean losing control over future treatment, or to the feeling that the team had already decided before listening. In such situations, additional medical explanation alone may not solve the problem. The team must ask what exactly lies behind the "no."

That inquiry may reveal a space of possibilities. A person unwilling to take one medication may agree to another; someone who objects to an injection may agree to a tablet; someone afraid of a high dose may agree to a trial period. Even if the law ultimately permits treatment without consent, the effort to locate a point of choice reduces the feeling that the person's entire body has passed into the ownership of the system. Autonomy is sometimes preserved in the small details that remain open.

It is also important to distinguish adherence from partnership. A person may take medication every day and still not understand its purpose or feel able to discuss change. A system may pride itself on a high rate of "compliance" and still fail to create treatment that can endure after discharge.

Partnership requires the person to know what they are receiving, what to expect, what alternatives exist, and what will happen if they request a change. Over the long term, treatment that a person understands and is willing to continue may be more stable than treatment that existed only while the door was locked.

Documentation is one of the quietest tools for protecting autonomy. When the record says only "the patient refused," the story behind the refusal disappears. When it records that the person feared a particular side effect, requested an alternative, received an explanation, and was offered another option, the file changes from a memory of confrontation into a record of a decision-making process.

That difference matters to the next team, to a reviewing body, and especially to the patient, who can see that their position was recorded even if it was not accepted.

The point at which the conversation is reopened also matters. A decision made and enforced during acute turmoil should not remain closed once the person stabilizes. The discussion can be reopened, alternatives offered, and the possibility of consent reconsidered. This expresses a principle of reversibility: the longer an infringement of autonomy continues, the more actively the system must look for the moment when the decision can be returned to the person.

Returning to the conversation is not only a legal matter. It also creates an opportunity to rebuild trust. A person may say that the treatment helped but the way it was given was difficult, or the opposite - that the treatment remains unacceptable even in retrospect. A system capable of hearing both possibilities makes clear that coercion does not turn the patient into someone whose voice has lost its significance; the person’s voice remains relevant even after a decision has been made against their wishes.

This separation preserves a fundamental principle: medical knowledge answers the question of what may help; law and ethics answer the question of when it is permissible to do so against a person’s wishes.

Chapter Twenty-Two

Restraint, Seclusion, and Restrictive Measures

Where Treatment Most Closely Resembles the Use of Force

Mechanical restraint and seclusion are among the most difficult interventions in the experience of psychiatric hospitalization. Even when they are used to prevent immediate harm, they can be experienced as a total loss of control, humiliation, and fear.

Discussion of these measures cannot stop at the question of whether their use is legally permissible. The modern question is how to reduce their use to the lowest possible level, and what a system must do to avoid reaching a point at which restraint appears to be the only option.

In 2016, the Israeli Ministry of Health appointed a committee to reduce the use of mechanical restraint. The committee submitted its recommendations in 2017, and in April 2018 a dedicated Director General circular was issued on mechanical restraint and seclusion in psychiatric hospitalization.

The circular explicitly presented reduction as both a clinical and a humanitarian objective and imposed stricter conditions together with supervision, oversight, and reporting. Its conceptual significance is important: restraint is no longer treated as a routine tool whose method of application merely needs regulation, but as an exceptional event that the system should work to prevent.

Restrictive measures should not be used as punishment, education, discipline, a response to refusal of medication, or a solution to staff shortages. The principle may appear self-evident, but it is essential because, in a closed setting, the boundaries between treatment, control, and discipline can easily become blurred.

If a patient raises their voice, curses, or refuses to cooperate, the behavior may be difficult for staff to manage. It is not, by itself, a justification for restraint. The justification must be the prevention of danger at the level required by law and professional directives, when no less restrictive measure is sufficient.

Can Zero Restraint Be Achieved?

The term "Zero Restraint" expresses an aspiration toward a system in which the use of restraint almost disappears. Some wards and systems around the world have substantially reduced coercive measures through organizational change. Even so, not every system or situation permits a simple commitment to absolute zero.

Restrictive measures lie at the most physical end of the coercion continuum. In involuntary hospitalization, the state removes a person's ability to leave; in mechanical restraint, it restricts the person's ability to move their body. Even when the decision is made within seconds because of a genuine fear of harm, it cannot be regarded as a merely technical act. For the restrained person, time may be experienced very differently. Minutes can feel prolonged, especially when the person does not know when they will be released, who is nearby, or what will happen next.

Staff stand on the other side of the same situation. A nurse or physician facing a person who is highly agitated, threatening, or harming themselves is not operating within a theoretical discussion of rights. They must protect that person, other patients, and themselves. Staffing may be limited, the environment may be noisy, and the decision may be made only after attempts at de-escalation have failed. A discourse that portrays every use of restraint as cruelty misses this complexity and may even alienate staff from the discussion. Reducing coercion requires acknowledging the fear and risk with which professionals must also contend.

This is precisely why the question must shift from "Was restraint permitted?" to the broader question: "How did the event develop to the point at which restraint seemed necessary?" Was the room crowded and noisy? Did the person ask for time alone when no suitable space was available? Did they try to explain that something specific was frightening them? Did staff know the person and how they usually calm down? Could medication, access to the courtyard, the presence of a familiar person, or a less stimulating environment have been offered? Sometimes the answer will be that every alternative was tried and proved insufficient. But asking the question itself turns restraint from an automatic response into an event from which the system is expected to learn.

A trauma-informed approach adds another layer. People who enter psychiatric services sometimes carry histories of violence, abuse, or loss of control. A physical intervention intended to keep them safe may recreate an earlier experience of helplessness. This does not mean that force can never be used. It means that staff should understand that a reaction that appears disproportionate may be connected to the meaning the event has for that person. Sometimes changing the way staff approach the person, avoiding sudden physical contact, or allowing the person to choose who remains in the room can prevent escalation.

After a restraint event, it is important to examine not only the medical documentation but also the experience itself. What did the person understand had happened? Did they know why they were restrained? Did they feel there was a point at which they could have calmed down but no one noticed? And what did the staff learn? A debriefing is not a trial of the employees and is not an attempt to prove that the decision was wrong. Its purpose is to turn a difficult event into knowledge that reduces the likelihood of recurrence.

At the system level, data matter as well. If one ward uses restraint far more often than a comparable ward, it is difficult to explain the difference solely by the characteristics of the patients. The difference may lie in training, staffing levels, physical design, staff culture, or the availability of alternatives. Measurement does not mean that every use of restraint is a failure; it makes it possible to identify patterns that are invisible when each incident is viewed in isolation. When data are presented to staff as a tool for improvement rather than blame, they can change practice.

The way staff speak to one another during an incident also matters. A frightened person may hear professional conversations taking place over their head as though they were not present. Short statements such as, "We are holding you so that you will not be hurt, and we will release you as soon as we can," do not remove the distress, but they keep the person within the human frame of the event. When all communication occurs in the third person, it becomes easier for the person to experience themselves as an object upon which others act.

These details are not marginal, because they are the materials from which the memory of a coercive event is built. A system seeking to reduce trauma cannot control every reaction, but it can control the way it remains present: by explaining, protecting privacy, providing updates, and returning to speak with the person afterward.

From the perspective of a person who has experienced restraint, the surrounding details are remembered as well: who spoke to them, whether their body was covered, whether anyone explained what was happening, and whether they were left alone. This is why standards must address more than the duration of restraint. Dignity during coercion is tested through language, privacy, and avoidance of unnecessary exposure. None of this makes a difficult event "good," but it can reduce preventable harm.

A genuine reduction in restraint and seclusion therefore requires more than an administrative directive. It requires adequate staffing, training in de-escalation, spaces that permit privacy, access to early treatment, and a culture in which an employee's request for assistance is not treated as weakness. A system that aspires to zero restraint is not claiming that risk has disappeared; it is declaring that every restraint event is exceptional and deserves examination of how the next one might be prevented.

One way to understand restraint is to see it not only as an event involving a patient, but as an event involving an entire ward. Before force is used, there is often a chain of interactions: workload, waiting, an unanswered request, a shift change, another person shouting, staff under time pressure. No single factor causes restraint, but together they can increase or decrease the likelihood of escalation. Prevention therefore requires a system-wide perspective, not only an assessment of the individual's behavior.

This approach also changes the nature of review. Instead of asking who made a mistake, the question becomes which conditions can be changed. Were there enough staff? Did anyone know the patient well? Was a quiet room available? Was the explanation given in a way the person could understand? Sometimes the conclusion will be that restraint was unavoidable even under good conditions. But reviewing every event creates cumulative knowledge and prevents the exceptional from becoming routine.

Staff well-being is also important. A worker who repeatedly experiences violence or threats may develop a heightened state of alertness that leads to earlier use of force. De-escalation training is important, but it is not a substitute for staffing, support, and conversations after difficult incidents. A system that wants less restraint must also protect those who are expected to stand on the front line. There is no contradiction between patient rights and staff safety; on the contrary, an environment in which staff feel safer can usually afford more time, flexibility, and patience before force is used.

Seclusion differs from mechanical restraint, but it too sharply limits the experience of control. A closed room can reduce stimulation and prevent harm, yet it can also intensify fear, especially for someone who experiences the environment as threatening. The question is therefore not simply whether seclusion is preferable to mechanical restraint. Both measures require justification, supervision, and continuous examination of whether they can be ended. Replacing one measure with another does not necessarily reduce coercion if the experience and duration of restriction remain equally severe.

Human presence is especially important here. Seclusion should not become the disappearance of staff. Even when a person needs a quiet and protected space, there is a profound difference between a door that closes them in alone and a situation in which they know who is checking on them, when someone will return, and what conditions will allow the measure to end. Information restores some predictability and sense of control to a situation in which most control has been taken away.

Reducing coercion also requires an organizational language that recognizes the event as exceptional. If staff speak about restraint or seclusion as a routine action during an ordinary shift, sensitivity to its meaning can erode. When every incident requires reporting, discussion, and learning, however, it remains present in professional awareness as something the system would prefer not to need. That culture is no less important than the written procedure, because in the end the decision is made by people under pressure and often within seconds.

The value of the goal lies in the way it reverses the burden of explanation. Instead of asking, "Why didn't you restrain the patient?" the question becomes, "What did we do so that restraint would not be necessary?" This is an important shift from a culture of risk management to a culture of coercion prevention.

Chapter Twenty-Three

Suicidality: Protecting Life Versus Autonomy

The Most Difficult Dilemma

Few situations demonstrate the tension between autonomy and protection as powerfully as a suicidal crisis. When a person expresses a wish to die, staff and family may feel that any mistake could be irreversible. The responsibility to preserve life pushes toward rapid intervention and, at times, coercion.

Even here, however, it is important to avoid an automatic equation: suicidal thoughts are not always identical to immediate danger, and danger does not necessarily prove that a person has lost all ability to make decisions. Clinical assessment must consider severity, immediacy, planning, protective factors, history, mental state, substance use, available support, and other relevant factors.

A health system is intended to protect life. When a person is in an acute crisis that narrows the ability to see other possibilities, intervention can allow time to do its work: the crisis may pass, treatment may begin, and a decision that seemed final in one moment may no longer appear so later.

This is one of the strongest moral justifications for intervention in situations of immediate danger. It does not rest on the claim that the state always knows how a person ought to live, but on the possibility that a temporary and treatable condition is closing off the person's ability to make future choices.

The danger is that the vital goal of suicide prevention can become a general rule used to justify every intrusion. Observation can be invasive; loss of privacy can be humiliating; involuntary hospitalization can deter a person from seeking help in the future.

Suicide prevention should therefore also be graduated and proportionate. There is a meaningful difference between a conversation and safety plan, intensive community treatment, observation, voluntary hospitalization, and involuntary hospitalization. The objective is to choose the measure that provides the necessary protection while preserving trust and liberty to the greatest extent possible.

A person who fears that any mention of suicidal thoughts will immediately lead to involuntary hospitalization may conceal them. A system seeking to prevent suicide must create a space in which difficult thoughts can be discussed without every conversation automatically becoming a coercive procedure.

This does not mean ignoring danger. It means distinguishing between disclosure of distress and a level of danger that justifies deprivation of liberty. The ability to make that distinction is part of professional expertise.

Risk assessment can never provide complete certainty. Staff act under heavy professional responsibility, but also within the limits of knowledge. After a difficult event, it is easy to judge a decision by its outcome. A professional decision, however, should be evaluated according to the information available at the time and whether the assessment was conducted reasonably and professionally.

A culture that punishes every risk may encourage defensive medicine in the form of excessive hospitalization. A culture that minimizes danger may abandon people who need protection. Achieving balance requires training, documentation, consultation, and services that make genuine alternatives possible.

Autonomy After the Crisis

One way to respect autonomy is to plan in advance. After a crisis has passed, the person can be asked what they would want to happen if a similar situation returns: whom to contact, what helps them calm down, which warning signs they recognize, which treatments helped, and which caused harm.

In this way, protecting life does not have to stand in opposition to autonomy. Sometimes the best way to protect a person in the future is to give them more control in the present.

This ambivalence helps explain why the conversation itself matters. Direct questions about suicide are not only tools for assessing risk; they may be the first time a person feels that someone can hear how unbearable things have become without immediately panicking or changing the subject. Sometimes the very possibility of putting the thought into words creates a small distance between the thought and the act.

At the same time, the conversation must not become a test in which the person learns what it is 'safe' to say in order to be discharged. If every disclosure is felt to lead automatically to deprivation of liberty, the incentive will be to conceal. A system that seeks early identification of risk must build confidence that not every suicidal thought produces the same response and that the intensity of intervention will be matched to the situation.

A suicidal crisis is not necessarily a stable and consistent wish to die. Many people experience ambivalence at the same time: one part seeks an end to unbearable pain, while another is still looking for a reason to remain. Sometimes the very act of seeking help expresses both voices together. A person who says, 'I cannot do this anymore,' is not always asking others to take over every decision; sometimes they are asking someone to help them through a period in which the available options feel exceptionally narrow.

Time has a special significance here. A suicidal decision may emerge within a window of hours while its consequences are irreversible. There is therefore a strong justification for temporary intervention when risk is immediate and the ability to see alternatives is severely narrowed. But the importance of time also limits the intervention: what was justified at the acute moment is not necessarily justified days later. Protecting life should not become an unlimited license to replace the person's will.

Risk assessment is not prophecy. Professionals examine history, planning, access to means, substance use, mental state, social support, and other factors, but there is no way to know with certainty who will attempt suicide and when. This limitation creates two opposite risks. Underestimation can end in tragedy; overestimation can lead to unnecessary hospitalizations and damage trust. A responsible system cannot eliminate uncertainty, so its decisions must acknowledge it: prefer proportionate intervention, reassess frequently, and use tools other than hospitalization whenever possible.

One important tool is a safety plan built together with the person. Rather than relying on the general instruction, 'If things become difficult, go to the emergency department,' it is possible to identify personal warning signs, people to contact, safe places, actions that reduce arousal, and ways of distancing dangerous means. The value is not only practical. The plan restores an active role to the person in protecting their own life. It says: even if a moment comes when you cannot see a way out, we can prepare a path now that may carry you through that moment.

The family has a delicate role. Relatives who have been exposed to a suicidal threat may live with constant fear and feel that they must supervise the person at every hour. A partner or parent cannot be turned into a private treatment team. Families should receive information, guidance, and a professional point of contact while the person's privacy and dignity are protected as far as possible. When all responsibility is transferred to the family, relatives are worn down and the person may begin to feel that every relationship has become a mechanism of surveillance.

After the immediate danger passes, a part of the work that often receives less attention begins: understanding what led to the crisis. Debt, separation, chronic pain, a sense of failure, loneliness, trauma, or worsening illness do not disappear merely because the person survived the night. Hospitalization can prevent an act, but it does not necessarily address the source of despair. Continuing care may need to connect psychiatry, psychotherapy, welfare services, social support, and sometimes concrete material solutions.

A conversation about suicide requires a delicate balance between listening and responsibility. If every expression of thoughts about death immediately produces the threat of hospitalization, people will learn to conceal them. If every statement is treated only as an exercise of 'choice,' the system may miss a situation in which the crisis has severely narrowed the person's ability to see alternatives. The quality of assessment therefore depends on a relationship in which the person can speak without knowing in advance that every word will be used against them.

Good risk assessment tries to understand movement, not only a static condition. What has changed in recent days? Has the person moved from a general statement to a concrete plan? Are they withdrawing from others, or actively seeking help? What is keeping them alive at this moment? Sometimes a small protective factor - connection with a child, a commitment to attend an appointment the next day, willingness to hand over a dangerous means - makes it possible to build a safer plan without hospitalization. In other situations, the overall picture may indicate a danger that cannot reasonably be managed outside a protected setting.

The intervention must not end when immediate danger declines. If the person learns that the only way to speak about wanting to die is to be taken to a locked ward, they may avoid the next conversation. After the crisis, the system should therefore return to the question of what might have helped earlier. Suicide prevention is not only preventing an act at the final moment; it is building a system in which a person can ask for help before a thought becomes a plan.

There is an important difference between an acute suicidal crisis and chronic suicidal thoughts. A person may live for a long time with thoughts of death without being in immediate danger at every moment. If the system responds to every disclosure in the same way, it can undermine the possibility of building long-term treatment. Patients quickly learn which words trigger emergency mechanisms, and some reduce what they disclose in order to preserve a sense of control. In doing so, the very information staff need to identify a genuine change in risk is lost.

It is therefore important to use a language that allows for degrees of risk. Clinicians can ask about the intensity and frequency of thoughts, planning, access to means, recent changes, and the person's ability to seek help. The aim is not to normalize danger, but to distinguish among different situations and allow a response that corresponds to the level of risk. When a person knows they can speak about a thought without hospitalization being the automatic outcome, the likelihood of genuine disclosure increases.

This balance also requires professional humility. Suicide risk assessment never produces certainty. Professionals can identify risk and protective factors, but they cannot know with certainty how a person will act. A good decision is therefore not one that guarantees an outcome; it is one based on the best available information, uses a proportionate measure, and builds follow-up. Acknowledging uncertainty is not an abandonment of responsibility. It protects against the temptation to convert every uncertainty into deprivation of liberty.

The discussion of autonomy during a suicidal crisis is therefore more complex than asking whether a person is 'allowed to choose death.' In most clinical situations, the practical question is how to protect someone while their ability to choose is narrowed without turning that protection into a permanent identity. Dignity does not always conflict with saving life. Sometimes it requires saving life in a way that recognizes that, after the crisis passes, the person will need to return to being the owner of that life.

Part Eight

Special Populations and Situations

Chapter Twenty-Four

Children and Adolescents

Autonomy That Develops with Age

Psychiatric treatment of minors adds another layer of complexity. In general medicine as well, parents make many decisions for their children, but as a minor matures, the child's own wishes and understanding carry increasing weight. In mental health, this is compounded by the concern that involuntary hospitalization during a sensitive developmental period may profoundly affect trust, identity, and the relationship with family.

The principle should be twofold: protect the minor from danger and severe distress while also recognizing the young person as someone with a voice, not merely as the object of adult decisions.

Israeli law establishes special mechanisms when a minor objects to hospitalization requested by the parents. According to current Ministry of Health information, when a minor over the age of fifteen refuses hospitalization, an application to the court is required; when the minor is under fifteen and objects, the matter is brought before the district psychiatric committee for children and adolescents. Hospitalization based solely on parental consent is also time-limited under the law.

The underlying message is important: a parent does not own the child's body or mind. Parental responsibility confers broad authority to protect and obtain treatment, but it does not erase the minor's wishes.

The reverse situation is no less complex. An adolescent may understand that help is needed and request treatment or hospitalization while the parents object. The older and more mature the minor, and the greater the understanding of the decision, the harder it becomes to justify giving no weight to that expressed wish.

The law recognizes situations in which the court must decide. The dispute then moves outside the family to an independent body expected to consider the minor's welfare, condition, and wishes.

Hospitalization of children and adolescents should be as brief and focused as possible, with a return to the community once it is safe. Children continue to develop while hospitalized. They need education, relationships, family, privacy, and a sense of future.

A child psychiatric ward cannot be satisfied with stabilizing symptoms. It must also consider return to school, relationships with parents and siblings, the young person's social network, and continuity of care.

In most cases, the family is a central partner in recovery. There are situations, however, in which family relationships are themselves complex and may even form part of the distress. 'Family involvement' therefore cannot be a blind rule.

Privacy, age, maturity, safety, and the best interests of the minor all need to be considered. An adolescent may sometimes need a private space to speak with a therapist even when the parents are deeply involved in treatment.

The Minor's Voice

For children and adolescents, the question of autonomy cannot be resolved simply by copying the rules that apply to adults. An eight-year-old child, a fourteen-year-old adolescent, and a seventeen-year-old young person are at different stages of cognitive, emotional, and social development. The ability to understand treatment, anticipate consequences, and express a preference develops gradually. The right question is therefore not only who holds legal authority, but how the weight given to the minor's voice should increase as the young person becomes more capable of understanding.

Family is almost always part of the treatment environment. Relatives can provide information the child cannot or does not wish to give, identify changes in behavior, and help continue treatment at home. The same closeness can also create conflict. An adolescent girl may fear disclosing self-harm if she knows every detail will immediately be passed to her parents; an adolescent boy may resist treatment because he experiences it as part of a family struggle. Confidentiality in adolescence is therefore not a luxury. It is a condition for creating a space in which the young person can speak honestly, while clearly explaining in advance the circumstances in which information will have to be shared to protect them.

Psychiatric hospitalization of a minor must also take account of the fact that development continues during hospitalization. Weeks away from school, distance from friends, and a sense of being different can shape identity at an age when social belonging is especially important. A high-quality setting does more than stabilize symptoms; it preserves, as far as possible, connection with education, family, and everyday life. Returning to school is as much a part of discharge as the medication prescription.

From the adolescent's perspective, the peer group within the ward also matters. Hospitalization brings young people into contact with others experiencing different crises and, at times, behaviors they have not previously encountered. A professional setting must therefore consider not only physical safety but also the social climate: how to prevent harmful imitation, how to enable supportive relationships without turning the ward into an alternative social identity, and how to maintain connection with the world outside.

The aim is for hospitalization to remain as brief a chapter as possible within development, rather than becoming the place where the entire process of growing up stops. Even when intensive treatment is necessary, attention must be paid to how the young person gradually returns to being a student, friend, and family member, not only a patient.

The inpatient environment itself must be age-appropriate. What calms an adult is not necessarily appropriate for a child. Staff need to understand development, trauma, family systems, and education, not only psychopathology. The use of force also takes on a different meaning when authority is exercised over the body of a minor. The younger the person, the greater the duty to explain, preserve contact with a safe figure, and seek alternatives that do not intensify fear.

There are also situations in which the interests of parents and child do not coincide. A parent may believe that a particular treatment is essential while a relatively mature adolescent consistently opposes it. Conversely, a parent may resist treatment the team considers necessary. The law must then balance parental responsibility, the child's welfare, the child's wishes, and protection from harm. There is no single formula for every case; this is why the quality of the process - listening, reasons, and independent review - becomes especially important.

Another sharp transition occurs when a young person moves from child and adolescent services to adult services. Almost overnight, a system that treats the family as a natural partner can become one that emphasizes the privacy of an adult patient. Young people can be harmed precisely at this point of transition. Good continuity requires preparation in advance: meeting the new team, coordinating medication, clarifying the family's role, and speaking with the young person about what they want to continue and what they want to change.

A further challenge appears within the education system. A school may be the first setting to notice a change in behavior, a decline in functioning, or concerning statements. It may also be the place the adolescent fears returning to after hospitalization. Appropriate communication between health and education systems should convey enough information to enable support without turning the diagnosis into information passed unnecessarily among staff. Returning to class often requires less 'explanation of the illness' and more straightforward planning around workload, examinations, attendance, and one trusted person at school whom the student can approach.

A minor's right to participate does not mean that the young person bears responsibility alone. The opposite is true. It means that the adults continue to protect the child while recognizing that this is a person developing toward independence. The way a system treats the young person's wishes during a crisis can influence whether that person will be willing to seek help from the system again in adulthood.

Consider a sixteen-year-old who arrives after an episode of self-harm. The adolescent agrees to speak with the team but asks that not every detail be disclosed to the parents. The parents, feeling that the ground has fallen away beneath them, demand to know everything. If the team shares all information, the adolescent may stop talking; if the team keeps everything confidential, the parents may be unable to help keep the young person safe at home. This is not an unusual case but an expression of the recurring tension in adolescent care: building individual trust without ignoring family responsibility.

A good solution is usually not found at either extreme. The team can agree in advance with the adolescent which information will remain confidential and which must be shared if danger arises, and can try to involve the young person in how that information will be communicated. In this way, even when parental involvement becomes necessary, it need not be experienced as betrayal. Transparency about the limits of confidentiality makes the relationship more predictable, and at an age when the sense of control is especially sensitive, that predictability has real therapeutic significance.

In children and adolescents, autonomy does not appear on a single day; it develops. A young child needs parents to make many decisions, while a seventeen-year-old may understand much of the medical information and hold a clear view. Law and practice therefore need to operate along a continuum, not across a sharp line on which the minor's voice has no significance before a certain age and becomes exclusive immediately afterward.

Family is part of the therapeutic environment and, at times, also part of the crisis. A parent can be the primary source of support but may also be exhausted, frightened, or in conflict with the child. 'Involving the family' therefore cannot be automatic. The system must ask who provides safety, what information should appropriately be shared, and what the child or adolescent wants. In some situations, another person - a relative, teacher, mentor, or regular professional - may be the figure through whom trust can best be built.

Hospitalization at a young age also affects development. Days away from school, separation from friends, and entry into the identity of a 'psychiatric patient' occur while identity is still forming. Community alternatives and preservation of connection with ordinary life are therefore especially important. The goal is not only to treat a symptom but to enable the adolescent to return to a developmental path in which the crisis is one chapter of life rather than the definition of life itself.

The education system is sometimes the first place where a child's psychological change becomes visible. Declining grades, absences, withdrawal, or outbursts may initially look like disciplinary problems. When school, family, and treatment services are disconnected, the child may move among competing explanations without anyone seeing the full picture. Appropriate information-sharing does not require full disclosure of medical information; sometimes a limited plan explaining what helps, who the contact person is, and what to do if the situation worsens is enough.

The transition from adolescence to adult services is another point of risk. A young person may have been known to a child and adolescent team for years and then move to a different system with new rules, clinic, and professionals. At precisely the period when greater independence is expected, continuity can break down. A planned transition should begin before the age threshold, include an introduction to the next service, and make clear who remains responsible until the new therapeutic relationship is established.

This brings us back to the idea of developing autonomy. The transition to adulthood is not merely a change in legal age; it is a process in which the young person learns to speak with professionals independently, understand medications, make appointments, and choose who may receive information. A system that lets the young person practice these skills before the birthday on which responsibility suddenly transfers strengthens the person's ability to manage future difficulties and potentially avoid crises.

The modern principle is not satisfied with hearing the minor as a symbolic gesture. The young person should be told what is happening in age-appropriate language, asked what matters to them, and have their position documented. Even when the final decision differs from the minor's wishes, recognition of the young person as a participant can change the experience.

Chapter Twenty-Five

Psychiatry and Criminal Law

Two Times, Two Questions

When a mental disorder intersects with criminal law, two entirely different questions must be distinguished. The first concerns the defendant's condition during the proceedings: can the person understand the trial and participate in the defense? The second concerns the person's condition at the time of the act: did the mental state satisfy the legal conditions that preclude criminal responsibility?

Confusing these two questions creates serious misunderstanding. A person may currently be unfit to stand trial even though they were responsible for their actions at the time of the event; conversely, a person may now be fit to stand trial while claiming that, at the time of the act, the legal defense relating to mental illness applied.

Section 15 of the Treatment of Mental Patients Law, together with the relevant provisions of criminal procedure, allows a court to order hospitalization or outpatient treatment when a defendant is unable to stand trial because of illness, subject to the conditions and procedures prescribed by law.

The question of fitness does not ask whether the defendant is 'healthy.' It is a functional question: can the person understand the proceedings to the required degree and communicate in a way that permits a fair trial? A criminal trial cannot be fair if the defendant is unable to participate in it at a basic level.

The second issue concerns responsibility. Israeli criminal law recognizes an insanity defense under demanding conditions. A psychiatric diagnosis is not enough, and even severe illness does not automatically eliminate responsibility. There must be a connection between the mental condition and the person's ability to understand the act or its wrongfulness, or to refrain from committing it, in accordance with the legal requirements.

The requirement of a causal connection protects against a stigmatizing assumption that a person with mental illness is not responsible for their conduct. Most people living with mental disorders retain full legal responsibility most of the time.

When a court issues an order for hospitalization or treatment within criminal proceedings, the mechanism differs from ordinary civil involuntary hospitalization. A significant amendment to the law in 2014-2015 established, among other things, a maximum period of hospitalization or treatment linked to the maximum term of imprisonment for the offense, together with arrangements for reviewing the defendant's condition.

The amendment was enacted partly against the background of cases that raised concern about the early release of defendants accused of serious offenses. It illustrates the tension between two approaches: if hospitalization is treatment, its duration should depend on medical need and risk; if it is tied to criminal proceedings, the seriousness of the offense also acquires weight.

The Israeli solution attempts to set a legal ceiling rather than require that the person remain hospitalized until that entire period has elapsed. Release within the period is governed by the review mechanisms and other provisions of law.

A fundamental distinction must be preserved: a person who is not criminally punishable because of their mental condition should not receive a 'sentence disguised as medical treatment.' The purpose of hospitalization is treatment and protection, not retribution.

At the same time, the public may find it difficult to accept the release of a person who committed a serious act once that person's condition improves. The moral weight attached to the gravity of the act can collide with the medical logic that there is no justification for continued confinement when the legal and clinical conditions for hospitalization no longer exist.

This is one of the settings in which law, medicine, and public emotion collide most forcefully. A rights-based solution does not disregard safety, but neither does it permit a hospital to become an alternative prison.

Committees and Review

Periodic review and reasoned decisions are important in the criminal-forensic pathway as well. The longer hospitalization continues, the greater the need to distinguish risk arising from an active mental condition from a generalized fear based on the person's past.

Criminal law and psychiatry speak different languages. Criminal law asks about responsibility, evidence, intent, and fair procedure; psychiatry asks about symptoms, capacity, risk, and treatment. When the two meet, concepts can easily become blurred. A person may be very ill and still bear criminal responsibility; another may be unable to participate in a trial even though their condition at the time of the offense was entirely different. Distinguishing fitness for proceedings from responsibility at the time of the act is a prerequisite for justice.

From the defendant's perspective, entry into a psychiatric-legal pathway creates a dual identity. The person is viewed simultaneously as a patient and as someone whom the criminal system suspects of, or has found to have committed, an act. Each role pulls in a different direction. Treatment seeks to build trust; criminal law relies on supervision, restrictions, and sometimes punishment. In a forensic institution, both worlds exist under one roof, and the person may struggle to know whether a conversation with a professional is intended to help or to assess dangerousness.

The public also stands within this tension. When a serious offense is connected to mental illness, a demand for protection naturally arises. But an exceptional case can shape broad policy toward many people who have never been violent. One consequence of automatically linking psychiatry with dangerousness is deeper stigma. Responsible policy must therefore protect the public without turning a psychiatric diagnosis into a general marker of danger.

Time carries a double meaning in this pathway. Psychiatric treatment does not follow the timetable of a criminal case; a person does not change clinical condition on the date a court has set. At the same time, liberty cannot be postponed indefinitely until treatment produces an ideal result. A line is therefore needed between desirable improvement and the minimum conditions required for release or relaxation of restrictions.

If the threshold for release is 'zero risk,' almost no one can meet it, because no person's risk is literally zero. Law must work with reasonable and proportionate risk rather than an absolute guarantee. This is especially important when professional opinions differ, as they often do in complex assessments.

The forensic pathway raises another question of time. In an ordinary criminal process, punishment is imposed within a framework tied to the offense. In a treatment pathway, the duration of confinement may be influenced by the clinical condition and risk assessment. This creates a danger that a person who committed a less serious act may remain in a restrictive setting for a long period because improvement is slow. This is one reason why statutory ceilings, periodic review, and a clear separation between the purposes of treatment and punishment are critical.

Victims and their families are also part of this story. A rights discourse that focuses only on the defendant can sound detached from the harm that occurred. Protecting human rights does not require ignoring the victim. It requires that the response to the act be lawful, proportionate, and based on the person's actual condition rather than on generalized fear of mental illness. It is possible to recognize the suffering of victims while also insisting that the psychiatric pathway not become indefinite imprisonment.

The language used to describe the person can also influence decisions. Over time, a forensic file tends to accumulate descriptions of risk, exceptional incidents, and violations. Everyday successes - months without an incident, consistent participation in treatment, a family relationship rebuilt - may receive less attention because they are less dramatic. Periodic review must guard against allowing the past to become a filter through which every current behavior is interpreted. Serious risk assessment relies on history, but it must also be capable of recognizing change.

The transition between hospital, court, and community is particularly sensitive. A person discharged from a forensic setting may need coordinated treatment, housing, and supervision. If the community is not prepared to receive that person, the absence of services can itself delay release. Once again, legal liberty depends on social infrastructure. A committee's conclusion that discharge is possible is not enough; there must also be somewhere to discharge the person to.

In the forensic hearing room, three different pictures of the same person may collide. The indictment describes an act; the psychiatric opinion describes a mental condition; family members describe an entire life that preceded both. A good system must be able to hold all three pictures without allowing one to erase the others. If only the act is examined, severe illness may be missed; if only the diagnosis is examined, responsibility and harm may be blurred; if only the life story is considered, current risk may be underestimated.

This difficulty explains why the forensic process requires genuine periodic review. The person today is not necessarily the same person they were on the day of the act, nor the same person they were on the day of hospitalization. Treatment can change condition, understanding, and capacity. Release does not erase the past, but neither can the past become a permanent hospitalization order.

The meeting of psychiatry and criminal law creates a unique tension because the two systems speak in different terms. Criminal law asks about responsibility, fitness, and protection of the public; psychiatry asks about mental state, treatment, and rehabilitation. When a person stands at their intersection, each system may see only its own question. The result can be that the person is viewed at one moment as a defendant and at another as a patient, but rarely as a human being moving between two systems of power.

It is especially important to distinguish unfitness to stand trial from exemption from criminal responsibility. The first concerns the ability to participate in proceedings in the present; the second concerns the person's condition at the time of the act. Confusing the concepts creates public misunderstanding and stigma, as though every person unfit to stand trial is generally 'not responsible for their actions.' The law requires a much more nuanced distinction.

The duration of confinement within a psychiatric-legal framework also raises a question of proportionality. A person who enters a treatment pathway because of criminal proceedings should not disappear into a gray zone in which rehabilitation and liberty are repeatedly postponed because the framework is complex. As risk declines and the person's condition improves, there must be clear routes for review, transition, and discharge. Otherwise, treatment can become an indirect form of punishment no longer connected to the original purpose of the process.

People in a forensic psychiatric pathway may also carry a double stigma: one arising from mental illness and another from their connection with the criminal system. The combination can make housing, employment, and relationships especially difficult. Rehabilitation therefore cannot begin only on the day the order ends. If the framework focuses for years solely on safety and compliance, discharge may arrive before the person has had an opportunity to rebuild a civilian identity.

This is why gradual transition pathways are important. Leave periods, protected community settings, supported employment, and follow-up can make it possible to assess functioning and risk outside the institution without moving in a single step from complete restriction to complete freedom. Gradual transition should not become a way to prolong restrictions indefinitely; it should be a tool for reducing them safely and on the basis of evidence.

Language matters here as well. A person who has been defined for years by the legal process through the act or the diagnosis may feel there is no way to escape the identity assigned to them. Genuine rehabilitation must recognize responsibility and risk where they exist while still allowing for change. If the system cannot update its picture when the person changes, an assessment that was once accurate becomes a permanent fate. Fair law and good treatment share a principle here: decisions should rest on the person's current condition, not only on the title of the case file.

The history of mental health law shows how easily 'temporary' hospitalization can last for years. Statutory ceilings, judicial review, and periodic hearings are therefore essential safeguards.

Chapter Twenty-Six

Life After Hospitalization

Discharge Is the Beginning of the Rights Test

It is easy to measure a mental health system by what happens inside the hospital: how long hospitalization lasts, which treatments are given, and whether the person is discharged. But the person's rights are tested no less on the day after discharge.

Is there somewhere to return to? Will the employer accept the person back? Can the person rent an apartment? Will information about the hospitalization remain confidential? Will family members once again see an independent person, or continue to treat them as someone incapable of making decisions?

Physical discharge from a ward is not always release from the label.

A person may leave hospital with a new diagnosis, medications, and recommendations - and with fear that the surrounding world will now see them differently. Stigma can affect intimate relationships, friendships, parenting, and employment.

The harm increases when the system itself adopts low expectations. If every ambition to study or work is regarded as 'too early,' rehabilitation becomes the preservation of stability rather than the construction of a life.

Work can be an important part of recovery, but it is also a setting in which disclosure of mental health information creates concern. Protection from discrimination requires distinguishing questions that are relevant to the job from curiosity or fear.

There are occupations and roles in which a particular medical condition may be relevant to safety, but even then assessment should be individualized and proportionate. A history of treatment is not equivalent to professional unfitness.

Workplace accommodations can make the difference between integration and withdrawal: flexibility during periods of treatment, a temporary reduction in workload, an adapted work environment, or support for a gradual return.

Housing

Without stable housing it is difficult to sustain treatment. Housing is a foundation for other rights: privacy, family, work, and community life. People living with severe mental disorders may encounter direct or indirect discrimination in the housing market and may sometimes depend on rehabilitation frameworks.

The challenge is to expand options rather than create a single pathway. One person may need a setting with close support; another may be able to live independently with occasional assistance. Rehabilitation should adapt the service to the person rather than force the person to fit the available framework.

A psychiatric diagnosis does not erase the right to intimate relationships or parenthood. Stigma, however, can enter family and legal decisions as well. When a child's welfare is being assessed, the focus should be on concrete parental functioning and safety, not on the name of the diagnosis alone.

Within the family too, control needs to be returned to the person. Relatives who played a central role during a crisis sometimes find it difficult to relinquish responsibility after the situation improves. The transition from protection to partnership takes time and may require professional support.

In an era of electronic information systems, psychiatric information may be retained for years and may be accessible to health professionals according to permissions and law. On the one hand, continuity of information can prevent errors and improve treatment. On the other, there is a risk that an old diagnosis will influence every new medical encounter.

A recognized phenomenon is diagnostic overshadowing: a physical complaint is interpreted through the person's psychiatric history, and the physical investigation is delayed or narrowed. This is both a problem of medical quality and a problem of equality.

The Right to an Ordinary Life

Ultimately, the purpose of human rights in mental health is not to create a perfect psychiatric system. It is to enable people to live lives in which psychiatry occupies the place that is needed - and not the whole space.

A person discharged from hospital should not have to prove every day that they are 'worthy' of liberty. Community life, work, education, relationships, and personal decisions are the person's ordinary civic starting point.

The next stage in the story is the new international phase: the United Nations Convention on the Rights of Persons with Disabilities does not stop at rehabilitation and equality within the existing model. It challenges some of the assumptions on which the model itself rests - above all, the possibility of using disability as a basis for deprivation of liberty and substitution of decision-making.

Discharge from hospital is a moment the medical system tends to see as an ending, but for the person it is often the beginning of the more complicated part. Inside the ward there is structure, medication is available, and professionals are nearby. Outside, questions of money, housing, work, relationships, and stigma all return at once. Someone who entered hospital with a job, a relationship, and a routine may leave to discover that some of those elements changed during the time away.

Returning to routine is not always linear. A person may work successfully for two months and then need a temporary reduction in hours; may begin studies and decide that the timing is still too early; may move to independent housing and discover that more support is needed. Rehabilitation that respects autonomy should permit movement forward and backward without treating every setback as proof that the entire attempt was a mistake.

The very possibility of taking one step back without losing everything encourages people to try. A rigid system promotes avoidance: if every attempt at independence threatens eligibility, a housing placement, or support, the safest choice is not to try. Flexibility is therefore not merely an administrative convenience; it is a condition for growth.

Returning to work sharpens the question of disclosure. Should the employee explain the absence to an employer? Request accommodations? Could a history of hospitalization affect promotion or the way every difficult day is interpreted in the future? There is no single answer for everyone. Some people prefer openness and experience it as a relief; others protect their privacy closely. The important right is that the choice not be forced by a system that circulates information beyond what is necessary.

Benefits and allowances can create a paradox as well. Financial support provides stability when the ability to work is impaired, but an abrupt shift between eligibility and ineligibility can make a return to work feel risky. A person who attempts part-time work may fear that, after succeeding for several months and losing support, the assistance will not be available again if the condition worsens. A good rehabilitation system should permit gradual experimentation rather than require an immediate choice between full dependence and full independence.

Housing is often the foundation for everything else. It is difficult to maintain treatment, work, or relationships when the place of residence is unstable. At the same time, rehabilitation housing can become restrictive if it dictates a person's way of life beyond what is necessary. The test is whether the framework moves the person closer to a life they have chosen or merely replaces a large institution with a smaller one. Privacy, the ability to host others, choice of housemates, and a reasonable degree of risk are all part of that question.

Social relationships change too. Friends and family can be sources of support, but at times they become excessively cautious. Every expression of anger is interpreted as deterioration, every unusual decision raises alarm, and the person feels continually watched. Genuine rehabilitation includes the right to become 'just a person' again - to be angry without every anger becoming a symptom, and to make mistakes without every mistake raising the question of whether someone should intervene.

The body can also be forgotten. People living with mental disorders need the same preventive medicine, examinations, and treatment for physical illness as everyone else. When every complaint is filtered through a psychiatric diagnosis, pain, fatigue, or another physical symptom may receive less attention. Genuine integration of mental and physical health is therefore also an issue of equality.

There is also a dimension of personal identity. After a first hospitalization, a person may wonder whether they are still the same person they were before it. Some rehabilitation takes place in conversations with professionals, but much of it occurs when the surrounding world stops relating to the person through the crisis. A friend who invites them on a trip again, an employer who gives an ordinary assignment, or a family member willing to accept a decision even when it is imperfect - all of these restore a place in a world not defined solely by treatment. This may be one of the hardest elements to measure and one of the most important to life.

Ultimately, quality of life after hospitalization is measured by the possibility of belonging. Not only receiving services, but being a neighbor, worker, parent, student, friend, and citizen. When a person remains identified first and foremost with the system that treated them, discharge remains incomplete. The purpose of rehabilitation is not to erase psychiatric history, but to return it to its proper proportions: a chapter in life, not the title of the entire life.

A small moment illustrates the gap between the ward and ordinary life. A person is discharged with a bag of medication, a summary letter, and a telephone number for the next appointment. From the hospital's perspective, the process has ended successfully. From the person's perspective, the questions are only beginning. Who will explain the absence at work? Does the landlord know? Who will be there on the first night? What happens if, three days later, thoughts begin to become unstable again but the next appointment is still two weeks away?

Discharge can be both joyful and frightening. On the ward there is a schedule, people are available, and the crisis is familiar to the environment. Outside, all the demands that were suspended return: bills, work, family, transportation, loneliness. A system that asks only whether the person is 'stable' may miss the gap between stability within a structured setting and the ability to carry the life waiting outside.

The weeks after discharge are therefore a test of citizenship no less than a test of treatment. Is there somewhere to live? Does the employer know how to allow a gradual return? Is there a community appointment? Has the family received general information about warning signs without unnecessary intrusion into privacy? Does the person know whom to contact at night? Every negative answer adds weight to the next crisis.

Stigma can appear precisely when treatment ends. A person returns to an environment in which people ask where they have been - or, conversely, avoid asking and keep their distance. The person must decide whom to tell and what to say. The right to privacy allows nondisclosure, but complete concealment can sometimes carry an emotional cost and prevent support. There is no single correct answer. A good system helps the person think through the choice rather than making it for them. Returning to life is not an appendix to discharge; it is where we discover whether treatment restored not only stability, but a place in the world.

Returning to the community also requires dealing with the mismatch between the pace of the system and the pace of life. A hospital can decide on discharge on a particular day, but a workplace may not be ready, an allowance may not begin immediately, and housing cannot be found according to the ward's timetable. Without coordination, the person may enter an interim period in which they are 'too well' for hospital but not yet connected to the supports needed for stability. That period can be especially vulnerable.

Good discharge planning therefore begins early. It is not a checklist written on the final morning, but a process of rebuilding bridges outward: contact with a clinic, medication, housing, social rights, family, and employment. Not every person needs every element, but everyone needs someone to ask what is missing. The more coercive the hospitalization was, the more important it is that the next stage be built in partnership. Otherwise, the person moves from the control of the ward into an unsupported void.

The right to community life also includes the right not to remain a 'patient' in every setting. People need places where diagnosis is not the central subject: work, a class, coffee with a friend, studies, parenthood. Sometimes the deepest rehabilitation occurs when the treatment system is present enough to support but not so present that it occupies the entire identity. The goal is not to turn every part of life into a service, but to allow services to recede gradually as life itself becomes stronger.

This is why 'continuity of care' is more than an administrative term. It is the connection between a place where the system carries almost all responsibility and a place where the person is once again expected to carry their own life. The sharper the transition, the greater the risk of rapid rehospitalization. A telephone call, a home visit, an appointment arranged in advance, or connection with a rehabilitation worker may look like small measures, but for someone leaving a closed setting they can be the bridge between discharge on paper and a genuine return to the community.

Part Nine

The New International Revolution

Chapter Twenty-Seven

The United Nations Convention on the Rights of Persons with Disabilities

2006: A Change in Perspective

On 13 December 2006, the United Nations General Assembly adopted the Convention on the Rights of Persons with Disabilities (CRPD). The Convention entered into force on 3 May 2008. Israel signed it in 2007 and ratified it on 28 September 2012.

The Convention is not concerned only with welfare services or accessibility. It seeks to change the way law understands disability: not as a condition that turns a person into an object of protection, treatment, or charity, but as a condition in which the person remains a holder of rights, will, preferences, and legal capacity on an equal basis with others.

In mental health, this represents a particularly sharp conceptual shift. For more than a century, psychiatric laws were built on the assumption that in certain circumstances psychosocial disability itself, together with dangerousness or treatment need, could justify deprivation of liberty and treatment contrary to the person's wishes. The Convention, and the interpretation given to it by the UN Committee on the Rights of Persons with Disabilities, cast doubt on the foundations of that model.

Article 12 of the Convention concerns equal recognition before the law and legal capacity. Its central idea is that persons with disabilities do not lose their status as rights-holders or their legal agency merely because they have a disability.

The implication for mental health is substantial. For many years, it was comparatively easy to move from diagnosis to the conclusion that someone else should decide. The Convention presses in another direction: before replacing a decision, support should be provided to enable the person to decide for themselves.

In its General Comment on Article 12, the Committee on the Rights of Persons with Disabilities emphasized the shift from substituted decision-making to supported decision-making. This position influenced legal reforms in various countries and also the development of Amendment No. 18 to Israel's Legal Capacity and Guardianship Law.

One important contribution of the newer discourse is the distinction between legal capacity and cognitive or clinical decision-making capacity. Legal capacity is a status: the right to be recognized by law as a person whose decisions have legal effect. Decision-making capacity is a function that may vary according to time, subject matter, condition, and the support available.

If the two concepts are merged, a temporary decline in decision-making ability can lead to a broad erasure of the person's legal status. If they are kept distinct, it becomes possible to seek accommodations and support without turning every difficulty into a loss of authority.

Article 14 provides that persons with disabilities are entitled to liberty and security on an equal basis with others, and that the existence of a disability shall in no case justify a deprivation of liberty by itself.

That formulation creates a profound controversy around psychiatric commitment laws. Many states argue that they do not deprive a person of liberty because of disability alone, but because of a combination of mental disorder with dangerousness or severe treatment need. The CRPD Committee, by contrast, has adopted a stricter position: when disability is a required element of the legal ground for detention, the structure itself is discriminatory.

The disagreement is not semantic. It asks whether the state may maintain two separate legal pathways: one for the population generally and another for people with psychosocial disabilities.

The Convention does not stop with liberty. It also addresses physical and mental integrity, the right to health, independent living, and inclusion in the community. Article 19, on living independently and being included in the community, is especially important to the critique of large institutions and to situations in which people remain hospitalized because no alternative is available.

The implication is that deinstitutionalization cannot mean simply closing beds. The state must build community supports - housing, treatment, employment, social support, and accessibility - otherwise liberty exists only on paper.

Precision is important here: the text of the Convention and the interpretation given to it by the Committee are not identical things. The Committee is a body of experts that interprets the Convention and supervises its implementation, and its views carry substantial weight in international discourse. Nevertheless, states, courts, and scholars do not always adopt the broadest interpretation advanced by the Committee, particularly regarding the complete abolition of involuntary hospitalization and treatment.

It is therefore inaccurate to say that the Convention simply 'prohibited' every form of psychiatric coercion in every country. It is more accurate to say that it created a new rights framework that led the UN Committee, the World Health Organization (WHO), and the Office of the United Nations High Commissioner for Human Rights (OHCHR) to call for a transition away from systems based on coercion toward systems based on consent and support.

This distinction matters throughout the book. The critique of coercion does not need legal exaggeration in order to be powerful.

In 2023, the World Health Organization and OHCHR published joint guidance on reforming mental health legislation. The guidance calls on states to build rights-based community services, promote free and informed consent, reduce institutionalization, and move toward ending coercive practices including involuntary admission and treatment, seclusion, and restraint.

This is more ambitious than the law in most countries. Precisely that gap is one of the most interesting features of current development: international normative standards are moving faster than national legislation.

Israel and the Convention

Israel ratified the Convention in 2012, after the Equal Rights for Persons with Disabilities Law and the community rehabilitation law had already been enacted, and before Amendment No. 18 to the law of legal capacity. In that sense, the Convention did not begin the Israeli transformation, but it strengthened it and gave it an international framework.

The Mental Health Treatment Law of 1991, however, remains in force. It continues to base coercive intervention on a combination of mental illness and additional statutory conditions. A tension therefore exists between current Israeli law and the more demanding international interpretations of the CRPD.

The deepest innovation of the CRPD is that it is not satisfied with asking how people with disabilities can be treated more humanely. It asks us to reconsider structures that permit decisions to be made in their place. In that sense, it moves the discussion from the institution to citizenship. A person does not possess rights only when stable, cooperative, or making choices that others regard as rational. The starting point is that rights belong to the person because they are a person.

Article 12, concerning equal recognition before the law, has become one of the Convention's most significant provisions for mental health. It strengthened the demand to move from mechanisms that replace a person's will to mechanisms that support the person in expressing will and preferences. The result is a philosophical shift: instead of asking who should decide 'for the person's benefit,' we ask how the person can be helped to decide for themselves. The distinction is not absolute in every situation, but it changes the default position.

Article 14, concerning liberty and security, generated an even sharper dispute. Some international bodies have interpreted the Convention as casting doubt on the very legitimacy of a coercive pathway grounded in psychosocial disability. Many states and professionals have responded that extreme crises may still require intervention over objection, particularly where immediate danger exists. The disagreement is not merely legal. It reflects two different conceptions of equality: does equality require abolishing a special pathway altogether, or may intervention be justified when it is based on risk and decision-making ability rather than diagnosis alone?

The Convention's influence can also be seen in the way it changes the point of comparison. In the past, improvement could be measured against the old institution: fewer restraints, more visiting hours, better conditions. The CRPD asks us to compare the life of a person with disability with the life of any other citizen. The question is not only whether conditions on the ward are humane, but why the person is there, what options were available outside it, and whether the person participates in decisions about their life. That comparison raises the standard expected of the system.

The Convention also links liberty to community life. It is impossible to speak seriously about reducing involuntary hospitalization if the person has nowhere to live, no support services, and no access to treatment. In this way, the CRPD brings the discussion back from law to policy. The right to liberty is not realized only in a courtroom; it depends on housing budgets, crisis teams, transportation, and services that can be received without leaving the community.

The CRPD generated unusual controversy because it does not confine itself to improving conditions within the existing model. The Committee's interpretation challenges the assumption that psychosocial disability may itself be an element justifying a special legal route to deprivation of liberty. For many lawyers and clinicians this creates a profound challenge: what is to replace mental health legislation when a person is acutely psychotic and poses a danger to themselves? For rights movements, the very framing of the question demonstrates how accustomed the system has become to thinking about people with disabilities under a separate legal regime.

There is no need to resolve the disagreement through a one-sided answer in order to understand its effect. Even countries that have not abolished specialized commitment legislation are now required to justify more carefully why distinctions are necessary, how they are narrowed, and what forms of support were offered before force was used. The Convention has shifted the reference point: what was once taken for granted has become something that requires explanation.

Perhaps the Convention's most important contribution is the change in the figure at the center of the discussion. Instead of a 'patient' who receives protection, it speaks of a person who remains a rights-holder even when extensive support is needed. The word 'even' is revolutionary: disability does not erase citizenship, and crisis does not eliminate every other preference. From that principle follow concrete questions about housing, rehabilitation, legal capacity, accessibility, and coercion - questions that connect all parts of this book within a single framework.

One concept clarified by the Convention is the difference between legal capacity and decision-making ability. Legal capacity is the person's status as a holder of rights and as someone capable of engaging in legal acts; decision-making ability refers to actual functioning at a particular moment and in relation to a particular decision. Conflating the two once made it relatively easy to conclude that a person who struggled to understand a decision had also lost the right to make it. The Convention insists on separation: functional difficulty does not erase the person's legal status.

That distinction does not solve every extreme case. There are still moments in which a person cannot communicate a clear wish or understand essential information. But it changes the starting point. Instead of moving immediately to substitute representation, the system looks for ways to support the person, interpret previously expressed wishes, and minimize the scope of decisions made by others. It is a small structural change in law but a large change in lived experience: the person remains the holder of rights even when assistance is needed to exercise them.

The family occupies a different place within this framework as well. Family members may provide crucial knowledge about the person's wishes, values, and history, but they do not automatically acquire ownership of the decision. The family moves from the role of presumed decision-maker to a source of support and information that must be balanced against the person's own will. In systems where family plays a central role, this is a cultural transformation no less than a legal one.

This tension is not unique to Israel. Nearly every country with modern mental health legislation is confronting it. The question is no longer only whether one clause or another should be amended, but whether it is possible to build a system that protects people in extreme situations without creating a separate legal pathway grounded in disability.

Chapter Twenty-Eight

Is the World Moving Away from Coercion?

There Is No Single "World Model"

Comparing countries tempts us to search for a winning model: which country protects rights best? In practice, mental health systems are too complex for a simple ranking. One country may have highly progressive legislation but too few services; another may allow broader coercive powers while maintaining strong judicial review and a rich network of community care.

Even so, several common trends are clear: limiting the duration of hospitalization, independent review, the principle of the least restrictive alternative, broader access to representation, advance care planning, a shift toward community services, and attempts to reduce restraint.

Alongside these trends, most countries have still not abandoned involuntary psychiatric hospitalization.

For more than four decades, the Mental Health Act 1983 was the central legal basis for mental health law in England and Wales. Long-running criticism focused on the use of coercion, disparities between population groups, the patient's status, and the person's ability to influence treatment.

On 18 December 2025, the Mental Health Act 2025 received Royal Assent and became law. The reform was designed to strengthen choice and autonomy, increase the patient's voice, reduce unnecessary detention, and alter some of the arrangements concerning people with learning disabilities and autistic people.

As of August 2026, however, precision is important: the new law has not yet been implemented in full. Some provisions have commenced, but most of the major reforms are intended to be introduced in stages. The government has announced that a new

Code of Practice is being prepared and that the first major implementation phase is planned for 2028-2029.

The British example teaches an important lesson: changing the statute is only the beginning of reform. Without workforce training, community services, operational guidance, and funding, new rights may remain for years somewhere between the statute book and everyday reality.

In the United States there is no single federal statute governing all civil commitment proceedings. Each state has its own framework, subject to constitutional limitations developed in federal court decisions.

Major decisions of the U.S. Supreme Court established that a person who is not dangerous and can live safely in the community may not be confined solely because of mental illness. The Court later held that civil commitment requires a standard of proof more demanding than the ordinary civil balance of probabilities.

State legislation commonly relies on grounds such as danger to self or others, but many states also recognize concepts such as grave disability - a severe inability to provide for basic needs - or serious deterioration. Some states also use forms of compulsory community treatment.

The American model illustrates the tension between relatively strong procedural protections and a fragmented service system. A person may enjoy significant due-process safeguards and still discover that treatment, housing, or support is unavailable in the community.

Canada likewise has no single uniform regime. Mental health law is primarily provincial and territorial. The grounds for admission, duration of detention, powers of treatment, and review procedures therefore vary from one jurisdiction to another.

In some jurisdictions the emphasis is on serious physical danger; in others, significant deterioration or forms of non-physical harm may also justify intervention. There are also important differences in whether involuntary hospitalization itself permits treatment without consent or whether a separate finding of incapacity to consent to treatment is required.

The Canadian Charter of Rights and Freedoms adds a constitutional layer of liberty, security, and equality, but it does not erase local variation.

Canada illustrates a point that is highly relevant to comparison with Israel: hospitalization and treatment do not have to be legally bundled into a single decision. A system can authorize the state to hold a person for a limited period while still requiring an independent legal basis for intervention in the person's body.

Australia: State and Territory Legislation

Australia also operates through separate mental health statutes in each state and territory. The frameworks allow involuntary treatment in hospital and, in some circumstances, in the community, together with review tribunals, rights to information, and in some systems access to representation or independent advocacy.

In recent decades, Australian legislation has increasingly adopted the language of the least restrictive alternative, supported decision-making, and advance planning. Coercion, however, has not disappeared. The gap between rights-oriented principles and actual rates of use remains a subject of research and criticism.

The Australian experience highlights the fact that inserting the words 'recovery' and 'least restrictive' into a statute is not enough. What matters is how those ideas shape day-to-day decisions.

In Germany, the Federal Constitutional Court has played a central role in restricting involuntary treatment and restraint. In a 2011 decision, the Court held that forced medical treatment of a person detained in psychiatric care constitutes a serious interference with bodily integrity and can be justified only under demanding conditions - including impairment of the person's ability to understand the need for treatment, use of the intervention as a last resort, and appropriate procedural safeguards.

In 2018, the Court also held that prolonged five-point or seven-point restraint constitutes a separate deprivation of liberty beyond the hospitalization itself, and therefore generally requires an independent judicial decision when it extends beyond a short period.

The German approach is instructive because it breaks coercion into separate components. The fact that a person has already been deprived of liberty does not give the institution an unlimited 'package of powers.' Each additional infringement requires its own justification.

In the Netherlands, the Wet verplichte geestelijke gezondheidszorg (Wvggz) entered into force on 1 January 2020. It replaced an older arrangement focused largely on hospitalization and permits several forms of compulsory mental health care outside hospital as well.

The law treats coercion as a last resort and requires services to offer voluntary treatment options in order to prevent it whenever possible. It is built around proportionality, effectiveness, safety, and the search for a less restrictive alternative. Courts play an important role in certain proceedings, and patients are provided with legal representation.

The Dutch model solves one problem and creates another. On one hand, it can avoid hospitalization by delivering care in the community. On the other, coercion itself leaves the hospital and enters the home and everyday life. The question becomes not only 'Is the person confined?' but 'How much control does the state exercise over the person's life even when the door is not locked?'

The Nordic countries are associated with strong welfare states and well-developed public services, yet they too maintain mechanisms of compulsory treatment.

In Norway, the declared principle is that medical treatment should be voluntary and that coercion requires statutory conditions and prior attempts at voluntary solutions, unless such attempts would clearly be futile or the situation involves serious and immediate danger.

Reforms in several countries in the region have tried to give greater weight to decision-making capacity and alternatives, but public and professional debate about the rate and use of coercion continues.

There is therefore no simple 'Nordic paradox.' Strong public services may create better alternatives, but they do not by themselves eliminate institutional culture or the use of authority.

The Comparative Conclusion

The world has not abandoned coercion. It is mainly changing the conditions under which coercion is permitted and the language used to justify it.

Three broad models can be identified. The first emphasizes dangerousness and permits hospitalization where danger is connected to mental disorder. The second adds tests of decision-making capacity and serious treatment need. The third, promoted by the CRPD Committee and by WHO/OHCHR, seeks to move away from a separate psychiatric regime toward a general system of consent, support, and rights that does not discriminate on the basis of disability.

International comparison also shows how dangerous it is to copy a single statutory provision from one country to another. A law operates within a system of courts, health services, professional culture, funding, and social expectations. A rule allowing relatively short detention can still be harmful in a country without rapid review, and may be more proportionate in a system where every decision is examined almost immediately. In the same way, a statute that speaks of a less restrictive alternative changes little if that alternative does not actually exist.

Systems also differ in how they understand the purpose of coercion. Some emphasize dangerousness; others give greater weight to treatment need and expected deterioration; still others seek to anchor will and preferences more strongly. These differences are not merely drafting choices. They determine who enters the coercive system: a person who refuses treatment but poses no immediate danger may remain free in one country and enter a compulsory pathway in another.

The data are difficult to compare as well. Rates of involuntary hospitalization are influenced by how 'involuntary admission' is defined, how events are reported, the structure of the system, and the availability of services. A low rate does not necessarily indicate a rights-respecting system; people may simply be failing to receive treatment. A high rate does not by itself prove overuse; the system may be recording coercion more completely. Serious comparison must therefore connect law, data, and the experiences of patients.

Culture also shapes the way liberty and support are understood. In societies where family plays a central role, a model focused exclusively on individual autonomy may overlook an important source of support. Yet heavy reliance on family can also obscure the person's own will. The choice is therefore not between family and autonomy, but how to build partnership in which relatives assist without becoming automatic holders of authority. Cross-national comparison is especially useful when it exposes cultural assumptions that we are accustomed to treating as self-evident.

The lesson for Israel is not to search for a perfect foreign model, but to identify elements that work: rapid and independent review, representation, accessible community alternatives, use of advance directives, transparent measurement of coercion, and crisis services that can be reached before the emergency department becomes the only gateway. A good reform can be distinctly Israeli and still learn from the world, provided it adapts the tools to the local structure rather than merely translating their names.

Comparing countries can easily become a competition in rankings: which country is 'advanced' and which is 'outdated.' In mental health, that is misleading. A statute that looks highly rights-oriented on paper can operate within a system that lacks community care, while a less stringent legal rule may function more proportionately where rapid review and real alternatives are available.

The system therefore has to be examined as a whole: law, services, courts, professional culture, and resources.

The data themselves require caution. A high rate of involuntary hospitalization may reflect overuse, but it may also result from a broader definition or more accurate reporting. A low rate can look successful while concealing people who receive no treatment at all. The important question is not only how much coercion exists, but who is subjected to it, how long it lasts, which alternatives were considered, and what people say about the experience.

This is the value of comparison for Israel. There is no need to copy the model of one country. We can learn mechanisms: how a review body gains independence, how a crisis service functions at night, how an advance directive is preserved and accessed, or how restraint data are published. Good comparison does not seek a perfect country; it breaks systems into mechanisms and asks which of them fit the Israeli structure. The world then becomes a laboratory of possibilities rather than a template to be copied.

Israel currently stands somewhere between the first and second models, while international rights discourse pulls toward the third. That gap is where the next reform is likely to take place.

Chapter Twenty-Nine

New Alternatives to Hospitalization and Coercion

Coercion Cannot Be Reduced Without Building Something in Its Place

The call to reduce involuntary hospitalization sounds persuasive until it encounters a person in an acute crisis at three o'clock in the morning. That is when real policy is tested. If the only alternatives are an unsupported home or an emergency department, the decision will repeatedly tilt toward hospitalization.

A rights-based reform therefore cannot begin and end with prohibition. It must build a continuum of services that makes it possible to intervene early, rapidly, and at different levels of intensity.

A crisis house is a smaller setting than a hospital, generally designed to offer intensive support in a more home-like environment during a crisis. In Israel, settings often described as crisis-respite houses or 'batim me'aznim' have developed in recent years, alongside similar models elsewhere in the world.

Their potential advantage lies in reducing the institutional experience, maintaining a stronger connection with community life, and building treatment in partnership. But crisis houses are not suitable for every situation. Where there is severe immediate danger or a complex medical need, hospital care may still be the safer setting.

The test is not whether every psychiatric ward can be replaced by a crisis house, but how many people who are currently hospitalized could have received a safe response in a less restrictive setting had that service been available at the right time.

Home Treatment or Crisis Resolution teams reach the person rather than requiring the person to enter an institution. They can conduct assessment, provide follow-up, adjust treatment, work with family members, and offer frequent support.

The advantage is that the person remains in their own environment. The team also sees the reality in which the person lives rather than only the person's behavior on a ward. It may therefore identify stressors, housing problems, or family dynamics that are less visible in an examination room.

The disadvantage is that home treatment requires substantial staffing and high availability. Without investment it becomes a limited service that cannot truly function as an alternative to hospitalization.

The Open Dialogue model developed in Finland and is based on a rapid response to crisis, network meetings with the person and people important in their life, continuity of the treating team, and a dialogical approach that tries not to fix one interpretation of the experience too quickly.

The model has attracted international interest because it emphasizes partnership and early community response. At the same time, inspiration from a clinical model should not be confused with the claim that every element has been proven uniformly in every system. Transferring a model from one country to another requires cultural and organizational adaptation.

Its central value for the present discussion lies in changing the sequence: instead of the system meeting the person only after the crisis has become dangerous, it tries to reach the person early and build a decision together with the support network around them.

A person in crisis may experience a professional as a representative of a system that has power over them. A peer worker with lived experience can sometimes build a different kind of relationship. Such a worker knows from within what it means to be a patient, to be hospitalized, to receive a diagnosis, and to return to community life.

Peer support is not a substitute for psychiatry or psychotherapy. It adds another layer of knowledge. In rights-based systems, people with lived experience are not merely recipients of services but partners in planning, evaluating, and delivering those services.

A crisis plan is written while the person is able to think calmly about what may happen in the future. It can include early warning signs, ways of calming distress, people to contact, preferred medications, treatments that caused harm in the past, and preferences regarding the place of treatment.

An advance directive is especially powerful in principle: it allows a wish formulated during a stable period to continue influencing decisions when the person's ability to express that wish is impaired. In this way it reduces the need to guess what is 'best' for the person.

Coercion can also be reduced inside the hospital. An open ward, where clinically appropriate, can preserve a sense of control and allow a person to leave and return according to agreed rules. Some systems have experimented with broader open-door policies even for groups who were previously treated almost exclusively in locked wards.

The issue is not binary. A ward is not rights-respecting simply because its door is open, nor is it necessarily harmful simply because it is locked. Physical liberty nevertheless matters, and every restriction on it requires justification.

Digital tools can assist with self-monitoring, reminders, remote consultations, and early recognition of deterioration. They can also create a new form of surveillance: monitoring sleep, location, activity, or telephone use can turn support into constant observation.

Technology is not neutral from a rights perspective. Future mental health policy must therefore address who collects data, to whom they are transmitted, and what happens when an algorithm flags a person as being 'at risk.'

The Real Alternative Is an Entire System

No single service can replace involuntary hospitalization. The alternative is a continuum: accessible primary care, a crisis line, a home-treatment team, a crisis house, an outpatient clinic, rehabilitation, housing, peer support, and hospitalization when it is genuinely needed.

The richer the continuum, the more possible it becomes to select an intervention that fits the situation rather than using hospitalization as the solution to every failure elsewhere in the system.

This is also the point at which the discussion returns to Israel. The question is not only whether the Mental Health Treatment Law of 1991 grants too much authority. It is also whether the state has created enough options for that authority truly to operate as a last resort.

The major challenge is not merely to establish alternatives but to connect them into a system that can be navigated in real time. A mental health crisis does not arrive with a label explaining which service will be appropriate. A person may begin with a telephone call, need an assessment at home that evening, and require a more intensive setting the next day. If every service functions as a separate island, responsibility falls on the person or family precisely when their capacity to navigate the system is at its lowest.

A continuum of services therefore also requires someone to accompany the person between settings. When a crisis team decides that home treatment is insufficient, it should know where the person can go and who will assume responsibility. When a crisis house completes its work, it must be clear who continues care in the community and when the next appointment will take place. And when a person leaves hospital, follow-up must not begin again as though there were no history. Continuity of care is, to a large extent, continuity of responsibility.

Availability is another condition. A service that exists on a list but is full for weeks is not an alternative to tonight's crisis. A service that accepts referrals only through a complicated pathway may be almost inaccessible to someone unfamiliar with the system. For an alternative to be real, it needs clear criteria, the possibility of rapid referral, and a response when the first service approached is not suitable. The test is not how many frameworks exist, but how often they could actually be used at the precise moment when the alternative was hospitalization.

There is also a danger that alternatives will gradually adopt the institutional culture they were intended to replace. A small setting can become rigid if every part of the daily routine is dictated from above; home treatment can feel intrusive when boundaries are unclear; digital monitoring can shift from help to surveillance. 'Less restrictive' is therefore not a permanent label attached to a service. It is an outcome that must be examined from the person's perspective.

The same setting may be liberating for one person and restrictive for another. That is why choice among alternatives matters, not merely the existence of alternatives.

A rights-based system seeks, where safety permits, to adapt care to preferences: treatment at home or away from home, greater or more limited involvement of family, in-person visits or remote contact, a short intensive setting or longer-term accompaniment. Not every option will be available in every situation, but the very effort to identify a preference changes the relationship. The person is no longer moved along an assembly line but participates in choosing the pathway.

Ultimately, alternatives succeed only if the system learns from them. It needs to know who reaches them, who is not accepted, who drops out, who returns to hospital, and what the user's experience was. If community alternatives accept only people with relatively mild conditions, they may improve service but may not truly reduce coercion. If, with sufficient support, they can also accept complex crises, they change the system's map of possibilities.

A good alternative is also judged by what happens when it does not work. If home treatment is insufficient and hospitalization becomes necessary, the transition should not be treated as a personal failure or as proof that the alternative itself was mistaken. A genuine continuum allows the intensity of care to rise and fall without forcing the person to start over each time.

A person may try a crisis-respite house, move to hospital if the condition worsens, and return to the community when possible. That flexibility prevents the system from thinking in only two categories: 'at home' or 'on the ward.'

Families also need choice. Home treatment always sounds less restrictive than hospitalization, but if it requires a spouse or parent to provide near-constant supervision without support, the patient's liberty is being purchased at a substantial cost paid by someone else. Alternatives must therefore assess the resources and limits of the household rather than assume that an available family is a free public service.

Location matters as well. An excellent service in central Israel is not an alternative for a person who cannot reach it during a crisis. Geographic distribution, transportation, and the ability to provide care remotely or at home are part of effectiveness. Precisely because small and flexible alternatives cannot always be located in every town, regional planning is needed to ensure a clear pathway in peripheral areas as well. The right to a less restrictive measure cannot depend solely on where a person happens to live.

The way alternatives are financed influences their character. A service paid only according to the number of days occupied may develop an incentive to keep beds full; a service funded only for preventing hospitalizations may prefer people who are easier to treat. A sound funding model should reward availability, complexity, and continuity, not merely volume. Otherwise, the goal of reducing coercion may conflict with the economic logic of the very services intended to make that goal possible.

Scale matters too. A small and intimate setting may succeed precisely because the staff knows each person, but rapid expansion can turn it into a small institution with the same culture it was designed to escape. Expansion therefore has to preserve principles, not merely a name: staffing ratios, real choice, flexibility, connection with the community, and the participation of people with lived experience in planning and evaluation.

Finally, alternatives need professional and public legitimacy. A family frightened for a loved one may feel that a crisis house or home treatment is 'less treatment' than hospital, even when it is appropriate and safe. Professionals will refer to a new service only if they trust it and understand how it works. Building an alternative is therefore also an exercise in building trust: through data, direct links with hospitals and clinics, clear criteria, and rapid opportunities for consultation. A service unknown to the people making decisions during a crisis will remain outside the pathway no matter how good it is.

In the end, alternatives should be assessed not only by the number of hospitalizations they prevented, but by what happened to the people who used them. Did they feel safe? Did they maintain contact with family and work? Did they return to crisis? Would they choose to use the service again? A system seeking to reduce coercion must evaluate the quality of the liberty it offers, not only the number of hospital beds it saves.

Part Ten

Israel Put to the Test

Chapter Thirty

Between Law and Reality in Israel

Rights Are Not Measured Only by the Statute Book

A country can draft a balanced law, establish review committees, entrench a right to representation, and declare coercion to be a last resort - and still create a reality in which a person's choices are sharply narrowed. The reason is simple: rights in mental health depend not only on what the state forbids itself to do, but also on what it makes possible instead.

A person in acute crisis who cannot obtain community care for weeks or months reaches the hospital system in a very different condition from someone who received help early. A family that does not know whom to call at night acts differently from a family with access to a crisis team. A psychiatrist working in an overcrowded ward with too few staff makes decisions under different conditions from a psychiatrist in a system with time, alternatives, and a complete multidisciplinary team. The question whether Israel respects the rights of people living with mental health conditions therefore cannot be answered simply by reading the Mental Health Treatment Law.

The test is systemic. It must examine the route from the first request for help in the community through the crisis, the gateway to hospitalization, conditions on the ward, the coercive process, rehabilitation after discharge, and the person's ability to return to a life that does not revolve around diagnosis.

The mental health insurance reform implemented in July 2015 transferred major responsibility for mental health services within the national health basket to Israel's health funds. Its aim was to connect mental health to general medicine and create continuous responsibility on the part of the health funds for both the physical and mental health of their members. In principle this was an important step: mental disorder should not remove a person from the ordinary healthcare system and place them in a parallel, separate system.

Demand for services, however, increased. Even before the Swords of Iron war, evidence had accumulated of long waiting times and staff shortages. After 7 October 2023, the need for mental health care expanded against a background of trauma exposure, bereavement, evacuation, prolonged reserve service, and disruption of ordinary life. The Bank of Israel's 2025 annual report, published in 2026, described an increase in the number of people seeking care even before the war and estimated a further rise in its aftermath. The state responded, among other measures, with a national mental health program launched in 2024 and funded with an annual addition of approximately NIS 1.4 billion.

That response deserves recognition. The mental health system of 2026 is not the same system that existed in 2015. Community services and alternatives to hospitalization have expanded; crisis teams, assertive home treatment, day treatment, crisis-respite houses, and psychiatric home hospitalization have been developed. The Ministry of Health now presents this continuum as part of the public response and emphasizes that in acute situations that are not life-threatening, alternatives to hospital admission should be considered.

But additional funding and the development of new services cannot eliminate overnight a shortage that accumulated over years. This is exactly where we must distinguish a change in direction from completion of reform.

Waiting times are often discussed as a managerial issue: how many days elapsed before an appointment, how many positions are available, and how many visits can be supplied. In mental health, waiting is also a rights issue. When a person waits for orthopedic treatment, the condition may worsen. When a person waits for mental health treatment, deterioration may also alter the degree of liberty available to them. A crisis that could have been stabilized in the community can become a situation requiring an emergency department, hospitalization, and even coercion. Access to early treatment is therefore part of a policy for reducing deprivation of liberty.

Public reviews over the years have pointed to prolonged waiting periods. A 2026 document of the Knesset Research and Information Center examining the mental health response after 7 October summarized earlier data according to which average waiting times for psychotherapy had in some periods reached months, while waits for an initial psychiatric assessment ranged in different places from weeks to months. The fact that the state had to allocate dedicated resources to shortening queues demonstrates that access is not a marginal problem.

At the same time, it would be misleading to present one figure as 'the waiting time in Israel.' Services differ, health funds differ, regions differ, and clinical urgency changes the order of priority. A national average can conceal both places where treatment is available quickly and groups that wait much longer. Serious policy therefore requires systematic publication of waiting times by type of service, region, age, and urgency rather than occasional estimates.

The Workforce: The Numbers Behind the Waiting Time

Availability of care depends on people. In recent years the State Comptroller has pointed to shortages of physicians in several specialties, including psychiatry. A report published in 2024 cited a 2019 estimate of a shortage of approximately 280 psychiatrists in hospitals and the community. Such a figure should be read cautiously because it reflects an estimate for a particular period rather than a permanent count, but the direction is clear: workforce shortages were a challenge even before demand surged.

The Ministry of Health's own 2026 work plan defines the number of psychiatry residents relative to the population as a national performance indicator and notes that a shortage of psychiatrists may delay diagnosis and treatment, lead to deterioration, and increase hospitalization. The choice of that indicator itself shows that the state recognizes a direct connection between staffing and system performance.

Even here, calling simply for 'more psychiatrists' is not enough. Modern mental health care rests on multidisciplinary teams: nurses, psychologists, social workers, occupational therapists, expressive and creative arts therapists, rehabilitation workers, peer specialists, and others. Shortages are not necessarily identical in every profession, but weakness in one link creates pressure on the others.

Workforce shortages also have a geographic dimension. A service that exists in Tel Aviv but cannot be reached within a reasonable time in the Galilee, the Negev, or a remote locality is not fully equitable. The right to health does not guarantee that every service will be across the street, but it does require deliberate policy to address distribution gaps rather than leaving them as an accidental result of the labor market.

Even when hospitalization is justified, conditions of hospitalization determine whether the deprivation of liberty remains limited to what is necessary or spreads into every area of life. Overcrowding, lack of privacy, high staff turnover, inactivity, noise, and a sense of having no control can deepen the experience of coercion even when the legal decision to hospitalize was itself proper.

The State Comptroller has in the past warned of exceptional overcrowding in some psychiatric wards and of its consequences for patient dignity, violence, and therapeutic capacity. Some findings relate to earlier periods and should not be presented as a uniform picture of every hospital today. The principle, however, does not become outdated: a system that seeks to justify deprivation of liberty in the name of treatment must ensure that the place in which liberty is taken can in fact provide treatment with dignity.

The issue is not aesthetic. Overcrowding and staff shortages affect the likelihood of escalation. When staff have too little time for conversation, de-escalation, and continuous presence, it becomes easier to reach restrictive interventions. Conditions of hospitalization are therefore part of a policy to reduce coercion, not a separate issue.

In recent years Israel has developed a much broader array of alternatives. As of August 2026, the government information database listed dozens of crisis-respite houses across the country, including general services and settings adapted to different populations. The Ministry of Health describes a crisis-respite house as an intensive service in a home-like environment intended to prevent hospitalization, and notes that it is designed for a person who agrees to treatment and can cooperate to a reasonable degree.

That last sentence matters. The very people at highest risk of involuntary hospitalization are sometimes those least likely to meet the consent and cooperation requirements of such settings. Expansion of crisis-respite houses, important as it is, therefore cannot by itself solve the problem of coercion.

Crisis teams attempt to close part of this gap. They are intended to reach a person in an acute state and provide short, intensive treatment in the community with the aim of stabilization and prevention of hospitalization. Psychiatric home hospitalization offers a higher level of treatment in the home, generally relying on the presence of a primary caregiver. Assertive Community Treatment (ACT) is intended to provide more intensive and sustained support for people with complex needs.

The next test of the system is not how many services appear on the Ministry of Health website, but whether they are available in real time. An alternative that cannot accept the person tonight is not an alternative to hospitalization that is taking place tonight. Measures of success should therefore include occupancy, availability, response time, the proportion of referrals that receive a response, and the proportion of hospitalizations prevented - while also preserving quality and safety.

In Israel, as in many countries, families carry a large part of the burden of community care. Relatives often identify the first signs of deterioration, help the person reach treatment, provide supervision during difficult periods, and support rehabilitation.

Some home-based alternatives even require a close relative or other person to serve as the primary caregiver.

Policy that relies on family must remember that not everyone has a family that is available, safe, or able to function in that role. Some families are exhausted after years of crises; some relationships are abusive; some people live alone; and some patients legitimately wish to keep certain information from relatives.

Family involvement should therefore be a tool, not an assumption. Confidentiality and the person's wishes must be respected, while families can still be given general information, guidance, and support that do not require disclosure of individualized medical information. A rights-based system does not choose between patient and family; it seeks to balance the patient's rights, the family's needs, and the system's responsibilities.

The Gap Between Discharge and Rehabilitation

One of the most sensitive moments is the transition from hospitalization back to the community. On the ward, the person is inside an intensive framework. On the day of discharge, they may return to the apartment in which the crisis began, a job that has been lost, debt, loneliness, or an exhausted family. If continuity breaks, the risk of returning to the emergency department increases.

Israel's Community Rehabilitation of Persons with Mental Health Conditions Law created an important infrastructure through the rehabilitation basket, but here too the question is availability and fit. A person does not always need 'a framework'; they need a precise combination of housing, employment, education, social connection, medical care, and support. Rehabilitation that does not take personal goals into account can turn from a pathway to independence into a new pathway of dependency.

Good continuity begins during hospitalization. The discharge plan should be built with the person, identify early signs of future crisis, establish a clear point of contact, and ensure that the next community appointment is not scheduled too far away. Here the recovery model and clinical safety meet: partnership is not merely a value; it may reduce dropout and improve continuity.

To know whether coercion is decreasing, it has to be measured. How many compulsory examination orders were issued? How many hospitalizations occurred without consent? How often were seclusion and mechanical restraint used? For how long? Are there differences between hospitals, districts, genders, and population groups? How many decisions were changed on appeal?

Data are not merely a research tool. They are a mechanism of democratic oversight. If one institution uses restraint far more frequently than a comparable institution, that is not automatic proof of failure, but it is a reason to investigate. If one district uses coercion more than another, the system should ask whether the difference reflects population characteristics, lack of alternatives, organizational culture, or the way authority is exercised.

Transparency should also include positive outcomes: crisis-team response times, rates of prevented hospitalization, continuity after discharge, satisfaction, and patient experience. A system that measures only beds, visits, and medications misses the question whether the person felt that treatment was done with them or to them.

The war that began on 7 October 2023 placed mental health at the center of Israeli public discussion on a scale that had not been seen for years. Broad groups required support: direct victims, bereaved families, hostages and returnees, evacuees, members of the security forces, healthcare staff, and civilians experiencing prolonged anxiety and trauma.

The system's response included additional funding, expansion of services, and development of community-based care. For the argument of this book, the change carries a broader meaning. When mental health becomes an issue affecting the public as a whole, the line between 'them' and 'us' becomes less distinct.

Stigma weakens when it becomes clear that a mental health crisis is not a characteristic of a separate group but a human possibility.

At the same time, expanding demand can deepen inequality if new resources fail to reach people who were living with severe disorders long before the war. A rights-based system must be able to respond to new needs without pushing the long-standing population to the margins.

The Law Operates Within the System, Not Above It

The central lesson is that good law cannot by itself compensate for a deficient system. A district psychiatrist may act cautiously, a committee may conduct serious review, and a court may protect liberty - but if no alternative was available before the person reached crisis, the range of choice had already narrowed.

This suggests a broader definition of 'last resort.' It is not enough that the doctor tried two options moments before issuing a hospitalization order. For coercion truly to be a last resort, the state must be able to show that it built a system containing earlier possibilities: accessible treatment, crisis response, home care, a community setting, and rehabilitation.

The gap between law and reality often appears in places that are not documented as a formal 'rights violation.' A person is told about the right to appeal but is too exhausted to understand it. A family receives a list of services but discovers that none has a place available in their area. A team knows that home treatment might fit, but the service is not operating at the hour when the person arrives. None of these events alone looks like a constitutional failure. Together they determine whether the choices that exist in law also exist in life.

This might be called rights at street level. It is where a statutory provision meets a queue, a staffing position, a bus ride, and an unanswered telephone call. In healthcare, and especially in mental health, those moments matter no less than court decisions. Sometimes the difference between voluntary and involuntary hospitalization, or between discharge and extension of detention, lies not in a new legal principle but in the availability of a service at the right moment.

A further test is regional variation. A right that can be exercised in central Israel but is almost impossible to exercise in the periphery is only a partial right. The same person, with the same clinical condition, may receive a different treatment pathway simply because they live somewhere else. National policy should therefore examine not only how many services have been established, but their geographic distribution, opening hours, and accessibility to people without a private vehicle or family support.

This is also why criticism of the system should be precise. Not every shortage is the result of indifference, and not every gap can be solved through legislation. Many staff members work under severe constraints and create solutions with considerable ingenuity. But precisely because their effort deserves recognition, we must ask which problems can no longer be solved through local improvisation and require structural change.

The gap between law and reality is often created in places that do not look like 'rights issues': an appointment postponed again and again, an exhausted worker who does not return a call, a clinic that closes in the afternoon, or a rehabilitation bed without an admission date. Each can alter the course of a crisis. When early care is unavailable, the emergency department becomes the gateway even for people who could have been helped earlier. In this way, a problem of access gradually becomes a problem of coercion.

The Israeli system has significant strengths: widely distributed health funds, a rehabilitation basket, public hospitals, substantial community experience, and newer crisis services. Precisely because the infrastructure exists, the next challenge is connection. A patient should not need to know which institution funds each service in order to receive continuous care. From the person's perspective there is one healthcare system, even if responsibility behind the scenes is divided between multiple bodies.

Public discussion should therefore move from absolute numbers to pathways. How long does it take from the first request for help to an appropriate response? How many people reach the emergency department after previously asking for help? How many are discharged without a coordinated follow-up appointment? How many alternatives are unavailable when needed? Data of this kind tell the story of rights better than the number of beds alone. They show where the system makes choice possible and where it narrows choice not because the law requires it, but because there is no practical alternative.

This leads to the next question. The Mental Health Treatment Law was enacted in 1991 - before Basic Law: Human Dignity and Liberty, before the Patients' Rights Law, before equality legislation, before the community rehabilitation law, and before the CRPD. Can it continue to be read through amendments and interpretation, or is it time to reconsider the structure as a whole?

Chapter Thirty-One

Is Israel's Mental Health Treatment Law of 1991 Still Fit for the Twenty-First Century?

A Law Enacted on the Threshold of a New Era

There is something almost symbolic about the date on which Israel's Mental Health Treatment Law was enacted. It was published in January 1991. A little more than a year later, Basic Law: Human Dignity and Liberty was enacted. In the years that followed came the Patients' Rights Law, the Equal Rights for Persons with Disabilities Law, the community rehabilitation law, the Convention on the Rights of Persons with Disabilities, and the amendment to legal-capacity law that recognized supported decision-making.

This does not mean that the 1991 law was already outdated on the day it was enacted. On the contrary, it replaced a framework dating from 1955 and sought to respond to criticism that had accumulated over decades. It reorganized powers, established committee and review mechanisms, and drew more detailed distinctions between different situations. In the terms of its time, it was a significant reform.

A law, however, does not live only within the year in which it was enacted. It operates within a changing constitutional culture. The question today is not whether the legislators of 1991 'were wrong,' but whether the structure they created still reflects the balance that Israeli society seeks in 2026.

It is appropriate to begin with what should be preserved. The law does not grant unlimited power to hospitalize a person merely because a mental disorder has been diagnosed. It sets conditions, regulates the authority of the district psychiatrist and hospital director, limits periods of detention, establishes psychiatric committees, and permits judicial review. In the criminal sphere it regulates treatment orders and the relationship between criminal proceedings and psychiatric care. It also contains provisions relating to treatment, rights, leave, and restrictive measures.

In other words, the law recognizes that coercion requires law. That principle must not be lost in any future reform. The answer to criticism of the statute is not to return decision-making to an unregulated clinical sphere. On the contrary: the more an intervention interferes with liberty, the clearer the rules must be.

The structure of psychiatric committees also reflects a sound principle: the person or authority that orders deprivation of liberty should not be the only authority deciding whether it continues. Independent review, even when imperfect, is a foundational element of the rule of law.

The most fundamental criticism comes from the newer international rights discourse. The statute is built around the category of mental disorder and, under specified conditions, permits deprivation of liberty and treatment without consent. The CRPD and the interpretation developed by its Committee raise a sharp question: may the law create a special route to deprivation of liberty specifically because a person has a psychosocial disability?

Israeli law has not adopted in full the CRPD Committee's more radical position that disability may not justify deprivation of liberty even when combined with tests of dangerousness or need. Like many countries, Israel continues to maintain specialized mental health legislation. But even without adopting the broadest interpretation of the Convention, the Convention at least requires us to ask whether every difference between psychiatry and other branches of medicine is truly necessary.

Why should a person with dementia, brain injury, delirium, or a physical illness that impairs judgment be treated under one legal framework, while a person with psychosis is treated under another? In some cases there may be clinical and practical reasons for different rules, but the mere historical fact that the systems developed separately is not enough to justify the distinction.

The Second Problem: Dangerousness as a Broad and Flexible Concept

The law uses tests connected to risk and mental condition. Every coercive system needs a threshold, but 'dangerousness' is not a laboratory value. It is a probabilistic assessment based on incomplete information, behavior, history, context, and professional judgment.

The concept carries two opposite dangers. If the threshold is too high, the system may avoid intervention until danger becomes immediate and severe. If the threshold is too low, unusual behavior, agitation, or a choice that others regard as unacceptable may be interpreted as a risk sufficient to justify deprivation of liberty.

Reform should therefore ask not only whether 'dangerousness exists,' but require a more structured explanation: what harm is anticipated? To whom? With what probability? Over what time horizon? What is the causal connection between the mental condition and the risk? Which alternatives were tried? Why is a less restrictive measure insufficient?

Requiring detail is not bureaucracy for its own sake. It forces the decision-maker to move from a general impression to a justification that can be reviewed.

The Third Problem: Decision-Making Capacity and Supported Decision-Making

One of the important developments in modern medical law is the move away from a global status of 'competent' or 'incompetent' toward assessment of capacity in relation to the particular decision. A person may be psychotic and still understand one particular choice; a person without a psychiatric diagnosis may lack capacity to make a medical decision because of another condition.

The 1991 law was enacted at a time when the discourse of decision-making capacity and supported decision-making was less developed. A future reform should therefore give greater weight to questions such as: does the person understand the information? Can they use and weigh it? Can they communicate a choice? And what can be done to improve their ability before their decision is replaced?

That last question is especially important. A person who struggles to understand a long legal explanation is not necessarily incapable of deciding; the person may need a simpler explanation, more time, translation, a trusted supporter, or a quieter environment. The right to make a decision is not only the right to be assessed. It is also the right to receive the support that makes decision-making possible.

The Fourth Problem: Rights Are Scattered Across Several Laws

A person hospitalized in a psychiatric ward does not live inside a single statute. The person is subject to the Mental Health Treatment Law, but is also a patient under the Patients' Rights Law, a person whose constitutional rights are protected by Basic Law: Human Dignity and Liberty, and sometimes a person with a disability under the equality law. If the person is entitled to rehabilitation, the rehabilitation law is relevant; if a supporter has been appointed for decision-making, legal-capacity legislation is relevant as well.

This fragmentation creates complexity. Staff members and patients should not have to be experts in five separate statutes in order to know what is permitted and what is prohibited. A future law could provide an opportunity to bring basic rights principles together in one clear framework: information, representation, communication with the outside world, privacy, consent, complaints, support in decision-making, consideration of alternatives, and protection from unnecessary restraint.

The intention would not be to cancel the general statutes, but to create within mental health legislation a clear rights gateway that a person can understand.

The Fifth Problem: Review and Representation Must Be Usable in Practice

A right to appeal is not enough if the person does not know how to use it. Someone in psychiatric crisis, confined on a locked ward, may be frightened, sedated by medication, distrustful of the system, or unable to read lengthy documents. In such a situation, the statement 'you may file an appeal' can be a theoretical answer rather than a practical safeguard.

Accessible legal representation is therefore part of the right to liberty. Yet representation also offers little real protection if it begins at the last moment, if the representative does not receive information in time, or if the patient does not understand the representative's role. A more advanced model should ensure that the person quickly receives a simple explanation of their legal status, the reason for the restriction, its duration, and the way to challenge it, and that they have effective contact with the person representing them.

There is also room to examine the structure of the committees themselves: independence, availability of members, frequency and timing of meetings, and the manner in which evidence is presented. The State Comptroller has in the past warned about difficulties in appointing committee members and about structural problems. If the committee is the gatekeeper of liberty, the state must invest in its functioning with the same seriousness it invests in the authority to order hospitalization.

The Sixth Problem: The Law Enters the Picture Too Late

The Mental Health Treatment Law naturally focuses on the moment when coercion is being considered. But a twenty-first-century system must ask what happened before that point. Did the person try to obtain treatment? Was there a crisis plan? Is there an advance directive? Can a crisis team come to the person? Is a crisis-respite house or psychiatric home hospitalization available? Can a short voluntary stay be offered?

A future law can therefore be imagined not merely as a 'hospitalization law,' but as legislation that imposes a positive duty to examine a less restrictive alternative. A decision to use coercion would have to record not only the reason for coercion, but also which alternatives were considered and why they were unsuitable.

This changes the burden of justification. Instead of requiring the patient to prove that treatment in the community is possible, the system would be required to explain why it is not.

The name of the statute also matters. 'Mental Health Treatment Law' emerged from the institutional language of its period: it defines a population and then regulates how the system treats it. The linguistic change that Israeli rehabilitation legislation underwent in recent decades was discussed in Chapter Sixteen; the important point here is the principle. Future legislation could begin from a different place - mental health, rights, and care - and make clear in its very title that the person is not merely the object of medical authority but a rights-holder within a treatment system.

A name, of course, is no substitute for content. A statute with a progressive title can remain paternalistic, and a statute with an outdated title can be interpreted in a rights-oriented manner. But the language through which law defines its subjects influences the way professionals and the public think about them.

Amend the Existing Law or Enact a New One?

There are two main routes to reform. The first is a comprehensive amendment of the 1991 law: updating definitions, strengthening proportionality tests, expanding representation, entrenching supported decision-making, regulating advance directives, and further limiting coercive measures. The advantage is preservation of a familiar framework and of case law accumulated over many years.

The second route is new legislation. Its advantage is the possibility of building the statute from the ground up according to a contemporary conception rather than adding layers onto a structure created more than three decades ago. A new law could begin with principles and rights and only then move to coercive powers - the reverse of the order that characterizes much historical legislation.

There is no purely technical answer. The question is how much conceptual change the existing structure can carry. If the necessary changes concern mainly details, amendment may be sufficient. If the aim is to move from a model centered on hospitalization authority to a model centered on autonomy, support, and the least restrictive measure, a new statute may provide a clearer framework.

What Must Not Be Lost Along the Way

The call for reform should not become an ideology that ignores extreme situations. There are cases in which a person faces an immediate and serious danger, the ability to accept help is profoundly impaired, and every voluntary attempt has failed. A society that refuses in principle ever to intervene may abandon precisely the most vulnerable person at the most difficult moment.

But that argument does not justify broad and unbounded power either. It supports a narrow, supervised, temporary, and proportionate emergency mechanism. The more the state claims that it is acting for the person's benefit, the more it must be prepared to show that it listened to the person, provided support, tried alternatives, and repeatedly examined whether the justification still existed.

An old law does not become obsolete merely because time has passed. Legal stability can sometimes be an advantage: professionals know the rules, courts have developed case law, and institutions have learned to operate within the framework. The mere fact that the 1991 law predates later rights legislation is therefore not proof that it must be replaced. The more important question is how much interpretive effort is now required to apply its provisions consistently with the rights-based world that developed after it.

Where interpretation and targeted amendments successfully close the gaps, there is logic in preserving the framework. But where central principles - the least restrictive measure, supported decision-making, advance directives, community rights, and transparency regarding coercion - remain outside the basic structure and have to be added from elsewhere, a different question arises: should exceptions and external interpretations carry the weight that the statute itself does not expressly carry?

Frequent legal change also has costs. Teams need rules they can remember and apply under pressure, and courts need a stable framework within which to develop interpretation. A new law, if enacted, should therefore be clearer rather than merely longer. It should bring together principles that are currently scattered across statutes, regulations, and case law, and present them in an order that can be understood even by someone who is not a lawyer. In a field where decisions are made at night and in emergencies, legal simplicity is itself part of rights protection.

Reform need not erase the past. It can preserve the review mechanisms built over thirty-five years, learn from case law and experience, and reorganize them around a different starting point. No longer a law that begins with powers and adds rights, but a law that begins with rights and defines the exceptions with precision. The change in order is not symbolic; it influences the way professionals learn the law and the first question they ask when a crisis begins.

The question whether to replace a long-standing law is not only legal. A statute is also an organizational language. For decades, forms, training, professional roles, and case law have been built around its terms. Comprehensive replacement can create an opportunity for new thinking, but also a period in which professionals are uncertain how to act. A good reform should therefore distinguish between what requires conceptual change and what should be preserved so that accumulated experience is not lost.

The 1991 law can be imagined as a structure that was well built for its time and has since received many additions. The question is not whether the building is 'bad,' but whether more floors can continue to be added without damaging its internal logic. When principles such as supported decision-making, advance directives, and the least restrictive measure remain outside the core, it may be time to redesign the structure. On the other hand, if those principles can be clearly entrenched through a comprehensive amendment, legal stability may be an advantage.

The choice between amendment and new legislation should be judged by results rather than symbolism. The test is whether a person and family can better understand their rights, whether professionals receive clearer rules in an emergency, and whether a reviewing body can examine the decision effectively. A new statute that is unreadable or unsupported by services may look progressive and change very little. Successful reform changes the sequence of actions in practice, not merely the order of sections.

This is the transition point to the next chapter. The question is no longer whether every reference to dangerousness should be abolished, but how to build a model in which dangerousness is not the final word. It is a model in which rights and decision-making ability do not enter the picture only after the state has already exercised force, but shape from the outset the way the system responds to crisis.

Chapter Thirty-Two

From a Dangerousness Model to a Rights-Based Model

Not Replacing One Question with Another, but Changing the Order of the Questions

For years, discussion of involuntary hospitalization was built around one central question: is the person dangerous to themselves or to others to a degree that justifies intervention? The question is important, and at times unavoidable. But it cannot carry the entire weight of the decision by itself.

A rights-based model does not abolish risk assessment. It changes the order of inquiry. Before asking whether force may be used, the system should ask what the person wants, what they understand, what assistance could improve their ability to decide, which alternatives exist, how urgent the situation is, and what is the least restrictive measure capable of achieving the goal.

Only after those questions does coercion enter the analysis. The change may look small, but its meaning is profound: the state does not begin with its authority; it begins with the person's liberty.

One of the central principles that should be expressly entrenched is a duty to choose the least restrictive measure. If the risk can be managed by a crisis team in the person's home, there is no justification for automatically choosing hospitalization. If an open ward is sufficient, there is no justification for locking the door. If a situation can be de-escalated through presence, conversation, and environmental change, the system should not move quickly to seclusion or restraint.

The principle does not require choosing the gentlest option regardless of whether it works. It requires selecting the option that interferes least with rights while still being capable of achieving the therapeutic and safety objective to an adequate degree.

This also matters over time. A measure that was justified in the first hour is not necessarily justified on the third day. The duty is therefore not only to choose correctly at the outset, but to keep asking whether the level of restriction can be reduced.

The least restrictive measure has two close legal relatives: necessity and proportionality. Necessity asks whether the intervention is truly required. Proportionality asks whether the expected benefit justifies the intensity of the interference.

In psychiatry, these tests must be concrete. It is not enough to say that 'the condition is severe.' The anticipated danger or harm must be identified, together with its probability, its seriousness, and the connection between the mental disorder and the situation. The decision-maker should then explain why the proposed intervention is expected to reduce the risk and why another alternative is insufficient.

The more intrusive the intervention, the stronger the justification should be. Forced medication, seclusion, and mechanical restraint are not merely technical extensions of hospitalization. Each is a separate interference with the body and with liberty and therefore requires a separate justification.

A rights-based model should move from the question 'Is the person ill?' to the question 'Can the person make this particular decision, and with what support?' A diagnosis is not the same as lack of capacity, and the severity of symptoms does not by itself answer the question.

Assessment of decision-making capacity should focus on four basic elements: understanding the relevant information, retaining it to the degree needed for the decision, being able to use and weigh the options and their consequences, and being able to communicate a choice. The precise language and emphasis vary between legal systems, but the principle matters: the inquiry concerns cognitive and decisional functioning, not compliance.

A person who says, 'I understand that the medication may reduce psychosis, but the side effects I experienced in the past are unacceptable to me,' does not lack capacity merely because the physician thinks the choice is mistaken. By contrast, a person who is unable to understand at all that they are in immediate danger may require a more intensive intervention.

Support Before Replacing a Decision

Even when decision-making ability is impaired, the immediate conclusion should not be that someone else must decide. Amendment No. 18 to Israel's Legal Capacity and Guardianship Law brought a broader principle into Israeli law: in some situations, instead of another person making the decision, the individual can be supported in making it themselves.

In mental health care, support can be very simple: a shorter conversation, repeating information, using clear language, allowing the person to rest before deciding, having someone they trust present, providing an interpreter, or involving a cultural mediator. In other situations, the team can rely on a crisis plan or advance instructions prepared while the person was stable.

The underlying idea is that difficulty in decision-making is not merely a characteristic located inside the person; it also arises from the interaction between the person and the decision-making environment. A noisy, threatening, fast-moving environment can reduce capacity. A calm and supportive environment can restore part of it.

Traditional medicine often spoke in terms of the 'patient's best interests.' This is an important concept, but it can become a screen onto which professionals project their own values. What is good for a person is not determined solely by the clinical outcome.

A person may prefer a medication that is statistically less effective if it allows them to continue working. They may choose a treatment that reduces symptoms less if the alternative causes severe weight gain or mental dulling. They may prefer to live with family even if the team believes a structured rehabilitation setting would be 'better.'

A rights-based model seeks to identify the person's will and preferences - not only at the moment of crisis, but across their life. When capacity is temporarily impaired, the system should try to reconstruct what the person would choose in light of their values rather than merely asking what a reasonable professional would recommend.

One promising tool is the psychiatric advance directive. During a stable period, a person can describe what helps in a crisis, which medications they wish to avoid, who may receive information, which hospital they prefer, what signs indicate deterioration, and which interventions have helped calm them in the past.

Such a document need not be an inflexible contract. Medical reality changes, and emergencies may sometimes require deviation. But a duty to consult the directive and explain why the team departed from it changes the balance of power. Instead of meeting the person for the first time precisely when they are least able to speak for themselves, the system encounters a voice the person left in advance.

Israel has room to develop a clearer legal framework for such directives: how they are stored, how clinical teams gain access to them, how much weight they carry, and under what conditions departure is permitted. Without an accessible mechanism, a document kept in a drawer at home cannot protect someone who arrives at an emergency department at night.

Early and Effective Legal Representation

Legal representation is sometimes viewed as something 'external' to treatment. But in proceedings that deprive a person of liberty, it is part of basic fairness. A lawyer does not decide what treatment is medically best; the lawyer helps ensure that the state complies with the conditions it has itself established, that the evidence is presented, that alternatives are examined, and that the person's voice is heard.

A genuine legal presence can also improve professional practice. When a decision must withstand real review, it is more likely to be written precisely and supported by reasons. Review is not the enemy of treatment; it is a mechanism that protects its legitimacy.

Reform should ensure representation that is early, accessible, and rapid. Consideration should be given to a model in which information about representation is provided proactively rather than only to a patient who already knows how to request it.

Judicial and Administrative Review That Is Not a Rubber Stamp

A court or psychiatric committee is not expected to replace the psychiatrist in making a clinical diagnosis. Its role is different: to determine whether power was exercised lawfully, whether the factual basis is sufficient, whether alternatives were considered, and whether the interference with rights is proportionate.

For review to be effective, the reviewing body needs enough information and cannot rely on general formulas. It should be able to ask: what actually happened? What has changed since the order was issued? Which alternative was examined? What does the patient say? What does the community treating team say? Does the risk still exist at the same intensity?

The central principle is that continued coercion cannot follow automatically from the fact that coercion was justified in the past. Every day of deprivation of liberty requires a current justification.

Reducing Restraint and Seclusion Through System Change

The Ministry of Health's 2018 directive marked a clear Israeli move toward reducing mechanical restraint and seclusion. But real reduction is not achieved simply by a rule saying 'use less.' It requires staffing, de-escalation training, an appropriate physical environment, analysis of incidents, and organizational culture.

Every restraint event should also become a learning event. What preceded it? Were there early warning signs? What did the staff try? What does the patient say might have helped? Did the physical environment or workload contribute to escalation? Is the same person being restrained repeatedly?

Sound policy should publish comparative data adjusted, as far as possible, for differences in patient complexity and set reduction goals, while avoiding the problematic incentive of 'zero at any cost,' which may simply displace coercion into less visible forms. The aim is less coercion in reality, not merely fewer recorded episodes of one particular type.

Culture, Communication, and Social Conditions

Coercion does not occur in a cultural vacuum. Behavior can be interpreted differently when the patient and the staff do not share a language, social codes, or religious understandings. A belief that seems unusual to a professional may be accepted in a particular community; silence may be interpreted as refusal to cooperate even when it results from lack of understanding.

Translation, cultural mediation, and training for work with different communities are therefore rights-protection measures. The more serious the decision, the less acceptable it is for it to rest on poor communication.

Social inequalities matter as well. Poverty, homelessness, substance use, and lack of a support network can increase the likelihood that a person will reach crisis. If the state responds to the outcome through psychiatric hospitalization without addressing the causes, psychiatric coercion can become a substitute for social policy.

Measuring a Rights-Based Mental Health System

A traditional system can be measured by numbers of beds, occupancy rates, length of hospitalization, and number of visits. All of these measures matter. A rights-based system should add others:

- How many crises were managed in the community without hospitalization?
- How many people received an explanation of their rights and understood it?
- How many coercive decisions documented the alternatives that had been considered?
- How much time passed between the first request for help and an actual response?
- How many patients participated meaningfully in their treatment and discharge plans?
- How many restraint events occurred, and how long did they last?
- How many people received follow-up care within a short period after discharge?
- What was the patient experience, including among people treated under coercion?

The measure of success is not whether the system 'defeated' the patient during a crisis. Success is that the person emerged from the crisis alive, with less harm, with more capacity for choice, and with a better chance of avoiding another coercive intervention.

Dangerousness as Part of the Model - Not Its Center

Dangerousness remains relevant even in a rights-based model. A society cannot ignore a genuine risk of suicide or serious harm to others. The difference is that risk does not define the person and does not release the system from its other obligations.

The change can be summarized this way: the old model asks, 'Are we allowed to stop this person?' The new model asks, 'What is required to protect life and safety while interfering as little as possible with liberty and will?'

The rights-based model can be translated into a relatively simple decision sequence. First, define precisely the risk or need rather than relying on a diagnosis. Next, examine what the person understands and what they want. Then try to strengthen their ability to decide through support. Only after that should alternatives be considered, moving from less restrictive to more restrictive measures. If coercion is nevertheless required, define its purpose, duration, and conditions for renewed review. When the event ends, return to the person and ask what can be learned for the next crisis.

The advantage of such a sequence is that it also supports retrospective review. Instead of asking only whether 'dangerousness existed,' the system can ask where the available options disappeared: was support unavailable, was no alternative available, or was the decision not reviewed soon enough? In this way, difficult cases can be studied without reducing every adverse outcome to a search for one person to blame. A learning system must be able to recognize both a reasonable decision that ended badly and a weak decision that happened to end well.

This sequence matters because it prevents the decision from becoming a shortcut. When the process begins with the word 'dangerousness,' it is easy to move rapidly to the tool the system knows best - hospitalization. When it begins with a series of questions, risk remains central but does not close the discussion. Sometimes the conclusion will be exactly the same: there is no safe alternative to hospitalization. The decision, however, will be more transparent, more reviewable, and more closely tied to the person's concrete situation rather than to a broad category.

A rights-based model must also be usable under pressure. If it remains a collection of attractive principles suited to academic discussion but too complex to remember in an emergency department, it will disappear precisely where it is needed most. There is therefore value in a simple order of decision-making: understand the situation and risk; identify will and preferences; strengthen capacity through support; examine alternatives; and only then, if the legal conditions are met, choose an intervention that restricts the person no more than necessary.

This order does not guarantee a 'softer' result in every case. Sometimes the end point will still be involuntary hospitalization. Its importance is that it requires the system to pass through questions that might otherwise be skipped. It also makes later review more meaningful. If no alternative service was available, the failure may lie not in the psychiatrist's judgment but in service planning. If no attempt was made to explain or support, the problem is different. The case can then be studied rather than reduced to a single question about dangerousness.

Such a model also changes measurement. A system would not be judged only by the number of hospitalizations avoided, but by the quality of the process: how many people received support before their decisions were replaced, how many alternatives were examined, how long coercion lasted, and how often the degree of restriction was reduced as the situation improved. Rights thereby become not an abstract concept but work indicators that can be observed, improved, and compared.

This is not semantics. The second question requires a richer, more critical, and in the short term more expensive system. But it may also prevent hospitalizations, preserve trust, and reduce the human and economic cost of repeated crises.

Chapter Thirty-Three

A Proposal for Israeli Reform

From Targeted Reform to a New Social Compact

More than three decades after enactment of the Mental Health Treatment Law, it is no longer enough to ask which individual section should be amended. Israel needs a broader discussion about the relationship between the state and a person during a mental health crisis. It is a discussion about power, responsibility, liberty, treatment, family, and community.

A proposal for reform need not begin from the assumption that everything currently in place has failed. On the contrary, Israel has a broad public system, legislation that permits review, a rehabilitation basket, developing community services, alternatives to hospitalization, and highly trained treatment professions. Reform should build on that infrastructure while shifting its center of gravity.

The proposed guiding principle is simple: consensual treatment in the community is the default; coercion is a narrow, temporary, and supervised exception that the state must justify not only by the severity of the crisis, but also by the alternatives it made available to the person.

Israel should consider replacing the 1991 statute with new legislation - for example, a 'Mental Health, Rights and Treatment Law.' The law should begin with a chapter of principles rather than a chapter of powers. The opening chapter could entrench the following principles:

1. Human dignity and liberty.
2. Equality and prohibition of discrimination on the basis of psychosocial disability.
3. A right to high-quality and accessible community-based care.
4. Autonomy and informed consent.
5. A right to support in decision-making.

6. The principle of the least restrictive measure.
7. A duty to preserve continuity of care.
8. A right to information, privacy, and communication with the outside world.
9. A right to legal representation and independent review.
10. A state duty to reduce the use of coercion in a measurable and continuous manner.

Only after declaring these principles should the law define the exceptional situations in which liberty may be restricted.

A Structured Threshold for Compulsory Examination or Hospitalization

A decision to order compulsory examination or hospitalization should contain a structured evidentiary basis. The law should require express consideration of five components:

1. A significant and relevant mental condition. Not every form of distress and not every unusual behavior justifies use of a special coercive statute.

2. A serious risk or clearly defined serious harm. The decision should describe the anticipated harm, the expected time frame, and the facts on which the assessment is based.

3. A clear connection between the mental condition and the risk or harm. The statute should not become a tool for managing a social problem that is unrelated to the mental health crisis.

4. Assessment of decision-making capacity and provision of support. Refusal alone must not be treated as proof of incapacity.

5. Absence of a less restrictive alternative that can be implemented safely. This should be a substantive condition, not a box to be ticked on a form.

A model of this kind does not abolish professional judgment. It makes the judgment more transparent.

A Real Continuum of Community Alternatives

For a legal duty to consider alternatives to be meaningful, the state must ensure a continuum of services in every district. Not every service has to exist in every town, but every citizen should have an accessible pathway to intensive care that is not a hospital.

The continuum should include multidisciplinary clinics, crisis teams, Assertive Community Treatment (ACT), day treatment, psychiatric home hospitalization, and crisis-respite houses. Night and weekend services also need development. Crisis does not occur only during clinic opening hours.

As of August 2026, Israel already has dozens of crisis-respite houses and the Ministry of Health presents a range of alternatives to hospital admission. This is a meaningful foundation. The next stage should establish standards for distribution and availability: what response time is expected from a crisis team, how many alternative placements are required relative to population size, and what happens when a service is full.

A Crisis Plan and Psychiatric Advance Directive

Every person with a history of repeated crises or involuntary hospitalization should be offered the opportunity to prepare a crisis plan during a stable period. According to the person's wishes, the plan may include:

- Early signs of deterioration.
- People who may be contacted.
- Treatments and medications that helped in the past.
- Side effects or interventions the person wishes to avoid.
- Preferred ways of calming or de-escalation.
- Preferences regarding the treatment setting.
- Instructions concerning disclosure of information to family members.
- Details of a supported decision-making supporter, if one exists.

The plan should be securely accessible to relevant treatment providers. During a crisis, the team should be required to review it and document how it was taken into account.

Beyond a clinical crisis plan, the law should provide a formal option for a psychiatric advance directive. Its purpose would be to allow the person to continue influencing treatment even when decision-making ability becomes impaired.

The legislation should define the conditions for preparing the directive, its validity, how it is recorded, and the circumstances in which clinicians may depart from it. Any departure should be reasoned and limited to a significant clinical or safety need that could not reasonably have been anticipated.

Such a tool connects two periods in the person's life: the period in which their voice is clear and the period in which others may have to make decisions quickly. It transforms autonomy from a principle confined to one moment into a relationship across time.

Automatic Representation in Significant Liberty-Deprivation Proceedings

When the state deprives a person of liberty, the burden of protecting that right should not fall on someone who is in crisis. Israel should consider automatic, early legal representation in significant involuntary-hospitalization proceedings, while preserving the person's ability to choose a different representative if they wish.

Representation should begin early enough to permit genuine preparation for the hearing. Counsel should receive access to the necessary information, meet privately with the patient, and be able to present alternatives. At the same time, the patient should receive a short, clear explanation of the process in a language they understand.

There is no need to turn every clinical decision into a legal hearing. But deprivation of liberty is not an ordinary clinical decision.

Strengthening Psychiatric Committees

District psychiatric committees play a central role in reviewing coercion. They should have sufficient staffing, a transparent appointment mechanism, and clear institutional independence from the authority whose decisions they review.

Service indicators should be established: time to convene a committee, rates of postponement, interpreter availability, extent of representation, and accessibility of decisions. A decision should explain in comprehensible language why continued hospitalization is necessary rather than merely reciting statutory conditions.

There is also room for orderly anonymous publication of important decisions or summaries, as occurs in other legal systems, in order to promote consistency and develop professional discussion.

A National Program for Continued Reduction of Restraint and Seclusion

Israel has already taken important steps to reduce mechanical restraint and seclusion. The next stage should be a continuing national program that includes:

- Uniform reporting of every event.
- Measurement of duration, not only the number of events.
- Post-event review with both the patient and the team.
- Regular de-escalation training.
- Adaptation of the physical ward environment.
- Staffing levels that make prevention possible.
- Publication of system-level data in a form that permits responsible comparison.
- Special review of repeated use on the same patient.

The goal should be consistent reduction to the lowest level compatible with safety, rather than treating absolute zero as the only target in a way that could encourage under-reporting or substitution of one coercive practice for another.

Measurable Standards for Access and Waiting Times

The right to mental health care loses meaning when care arrives only after the crisis has worsened. Measurable waiting-time standards should therefore be established by type of service and urgency.

Routine psychotherapy and urgent psychiatric assessment do not need to share the same target. A graded framework is needed: emergency response, urgent assessment, psychiatric evaluation, multidisciplinary care, psychotherapy, and rehabilitation. Each area should have an appropriate target and periodic public reporting of performance.

Measurement should begin on the day the person requested help, not on the day the system formally opened a case. Otherwise, statistics can improve without the patient's experience improving.

Workforce as a Rights Infrastructure

There is no rights reform without a workforce. If a psychiatrist is responsible for more patients than can reasonably be treated, if a nurse on a ward is responsible for more people than can safely be observed, or if a social worker has no time for discharge planning, rights erode even when no one intends them to.

The state should continue expanding training and specialist pathways in adult psychiatry and child and adolescent psychiatry, but it must also build a multidisciplinary workforce plan. That plan should address the periphery, burnout, and staff retention, not merely the number of posts on paper.

Peer specialists with lived experience deserve particular attention. Their inclusion in clinical teams, training, and planning committees can contribute a form of knowledge that a professional system alone does not possess.

Open Data and Transparency

The Ministry of Health already publishes data and statistical yearbooks, but reform could broaden transparency through a regularly updated public dashboard containing, without identifying patients:

- Voluntary and involuntary hospitalizations.
- Length of hospitalization.
- Use of seclusion and mechanical restraint.
- Waiting times.
- Activity of crisis teams and psychiatric home hospitalization.
- Availability of crisis-respite houses.
- Continuity of care after discharge.
- Patient-experience and complaint indicators.
- Regional and demographic disparities.

Transparency is not intended to shame institutions. It allows variation to be identified, lessons to be learned from places that perform well, and resources to be directed to areas that need change.

Hospitals and health funds are measured on many clinical indicators. Rights indicators should be added as an integral part of quality measurement. Examples include the proportion of patients who report participating in their treatment plan, the proportion who received explanations in understandable language, the ability to maintain contact with family according to the patient's wishes, and the proportion of discharge plans coordinated with community services.

The managerial message should be clear: dignity and autonomy are not a 'soft' addition after medical treatment has finished. They are part of the quality of treatment itself.

Families, Children, and Professional Culture

Families need more guidance, support, and access to professionals, especially during crises. Expanding their role, however, should not come at the expense of confidentiality and the autonomy of an adult patient.

A mechanism can be established in which each patient is asked in advance what information may be shared, with whom, and under which circumstances. Even when there is no consent to disclose individualized medical information, families can still receive general information about services, emergency signs, and appropriate courses of action.

Where the family is part of the problem, the system must recognize this rather than automatically assuming that relatives are the correct source of support.

Minors require a special framework balancing parental responsibility, the child's developing capacity, and the child's own wishes. The duty to hear the child or adolescent according to age and understanding should be strengthened, the process should be explained to them, and non-hospital alternatives should be examined wherever this can be done safely.

Community and family-based services for children should be expanded, because hospitalization at a young age affects education, relationships, and identity during a particularly sensitive period.

Legislation can establish boundaries, but it cannot create partnership by itself. A system can comply with every formal section and still leave a person feeling humiliated and voiceless. The deeper change depends on professional culture.

Training of mental health professionals should include not only diagnosis and medication, but also human rights, trauma caused by coercion, de-escalation, shared decision-making, work with peer specialists, and communication with families. Staff should systematically hear the experiences of people who have undergone hospitalization, including those who describe it as life-saving and those who describe it as a profound harm.

There is no single story of psychiatric hospitalization. Some people say, 'Coercion saved my life,' while others say, 'It broke my trust for years.' A mature system must be able to hear both voices without dismissing either.

A Possible Israel of 2036

Imagine Israel in 2036. A person begins to deteriorate and receives a response within hours from a team that knows the person's crisis plan. The person can choose a supporter. If intensive care is needed, several community alternatives are offered. If involuntary hospitalization nevertheless becomes necessary, the decision is reasoned, representation is activated quickly, and a committee examines alternatives within a short time. Restraint is rarely used on the ward, and every event is reviewed. Discharge planning begins at the start of hospitalization, and the transition back to the community takes place without a break in continuity of care.

The vision does not promise a world without crises, risk, or difficult decisions. It promises that the system will not use difficulty as a reason to abandon rights.

Not Less Treatment - Treatment With Less Force

Public debate sometimes presents a false choice: either protect rights or allow professionals to treat. But the purpose of reform is not to weaken treatment. It is to make treatment more legitimate, more precise, and more effective.

Good reform also cannot happen in a single day. If the law requires a less restrictive alternative before the state has actually built such alternatives, professionals will be left with a duty they cannot fulfill. If beds are reduced before crisis services expand, the burden will move to emergency departments and families. If supported decision-making is declared without training staff, the concept will remain on paper. Change must therefore be phased: legislation, budget, training, services, and measurement must move forward together.

Success should also be defined in advance. It is not enough to say that the goal is 'less coercion.' The system needs to know whether the number of involuntary hospitalizations declined, whether their duration shortened, whether restraint events decreased, whether more people received a community alternative, whether waiting times improved, and whether people themselves report greater partnership and dignity.

Such indicators also make it possible to identify unintended effects. A decline in hospitalization is not an achievement if more people are simultaneously left without treatment.

Phased implementation also allows the system to learn what works before expanding it. Reform can begin in areas where infrastructure already exists, measure the impact of alternatives, correct failures, and then expand. Such an approach is less dramatic than announcing a 'revolution,' but it fits a field in which every change touches people at their most vulnerable moments. The aim is not a reform that looks innovative on paper, but a system that works on Saturday night, in the periphery, and when a crisis is complex and does not fit neatly into the criteria of a single service.

Israel's advantage is that its healthcare system is not starting from zero. There is already a statute, psychiatric committees, community care, a rehabilitation basket, health funds, crisis-respite houses, home treatment, and crisis teams. Reform does not need to invent an entirely new system; it needs to connect parts that already exist and change their order of priority. That is the practical path for turning the principle of coercion as a last resort from an ethical aspiration into an organizational reality.

A broad reform needs priorities if it is not to become diffuse. The first stage should be the creation of infrastructure that makes it possible to demand less coercion without leaving professionals and families with no alternative. Only once crisis teams, community settings, and the ability to coordinate follow-up care are genuinely available can the duty to choose the least restrictive measure be tightened effectively. Law and services must advance together; otherwise each will place on the other a responsibility it cannot fulfill.

The second stage is to build accountability mechanisms. Each body should know what it is measured on: hospitals on restraint, patient experience, and discharge planning; health funds on response times and continuity; the state on geographic distribution and workforce; and committees on the speed and quality of review. Indicators do not replace professional judgment, but they prevent a situation in which everyone supports rights in principle and no one is accountable for whether they exist in daily practice.

The third stage is continuous public learning. Mental health reform will also produce unexpected results. One alternative may work well in one region and less well in another; a rule intended to reduce restraint may generate another form of restriction; expansion of a service may reveal demand that had never previously been measured. A mature system does not conceal such findings in order to protect the reform. It publishes them, examines them, and adjusts. If rights are part of treatment quality, failure to uphold them should also be data from which the system learns, not only a legal claim raised after a crisis.

Force can save lives in an extreme moment. But a system that relies on it too much pays in trust, cooperation, and harm. The challenge for the next generation is neither to remove psychiatry from law nor to remove law from psychiatry. It is to build a system in which professional treatment and human rights strengthen one another.

Conclusion - The Right to Remain a Person Even in a Moment of Crisis

This book began with a question that appears simple: who decides what is good for a person when their mental state becomes unstable? As we moved more deeply into history, law, and the everyday life of mental health systems, it became clear that there is no single answer. Sometimes a person remains able to decide even when others disagree with the decision. Sometimes decision-making ability is temporarily and profoundly impaired. Sometimes a family sees a danger that a professional has not yet recognized, and sometimes those closest to the person find it difficult to allow a choice different from their own. Sometimes coercive intervention prevents catastrophe, and sometimes it leaves a wound that makes the person less willing to seek help in the future. This complexity is not a reason to abandon principles. It is the reason to formulate them more carefully.

The historical journey shows how dramatically the point of view has changed. In earlier periods, a person whose behavior appeared unusual might be seen as sinful, cursed, or threatening. The birth of psychiatry changed the language: suffering gradually became illness, and the person became a patient. This was an enormous humanistic achievement. The possibility of seeing mental distress as a medical condition rather than a moral defect opened a path to treatment, compassion, and research. But it also opened another door: if illness can impair judgment, those who possess medical knowledge may come to believe that they are entitled to decide in the person's place.

This was the context in which large institutions developed. Some were created from a genuine desire to protect and treat, but as they expanded they sometimes became entire worlds in which order, discipline, and treatment merged. A person might lose not only the freedom to leave, but also the ability to decide how the day would look. The institution could provide shelter, food, and treatment while simultaneously narrowing identity, privacy, and initiative. The lesson is not that every institution is necessarily oppressive, but that a system that holds a person for long periods tends to accumulate power even when its intentions are benevolent.

The twentieth century brought new medical hope. Biological treatments, medication, and new therapeutic approaches changed millions of lives. In many cases they made it possible for people to leave institutions and live in the community. But the progress itself sharpened the question of consent. The more convinced the system became that it possessed an effective treatment, the easier it was to view refusal as an obstacle to overcome. From this point emerged one of the central debates of modern psychiatry: does better professional knowledge confer a right to replace a person's will, or does it instead create a greater responsibility to explain, involve, and justify every departure from consent?

Law entered this tension gradually. At first, it gave coercion a framework; later, it also became a means of limiting coercion. Courts began to require a medical foundation, dangerousness or a defined need, fair procedure, and review. The simple idea that 'the doctor knows best' was no longer sufficient on its own. Deprivation of liberty became an act requiring legal authority, reasons, and repeated reconsideration. The relationship between psychiatry and the state therefore changed: treatment remained a medical matter, but the power to control a person's movement became unmistakably a legal one.

Deinstitutionalization added the social lesson. A country can open the gates of the hospital and still fail to create liberty. A person without housing, income, accessible treatment, or social connection can move from the institution to instability, imprisonment, or repeated hospitalizations. The right to live in the community is therefore more than a right not to be confined. It requires real conditions that make community life possible. Housing, employment, rehabilitation, and community services are not 'soft' additions to the hospital system; they are part of the infrastructure that makes it possible to reduce coercion.

Israel followed a parallel but distinctive path. The 1955 law reflected the spirit of its period and the needs of a young state trying to regulate a sensitive field. The 1991 law created more detailed mechanisms, established review, and defined powers and procedures. Yet it was enacted immediately before a series of developments that transformed the language of rights in Israel: Basic Law: Human Dignity and Liberty, the Patients' Rights Law, the Equal Rights for Persons with Disabilities Law, the community rehabilitation law, and recognition of supported decision-making. In retrospect, the 1991 law therefore looks like a law of transition. It is not simply an old law, but it was written within a conceptual world that preceded some of the principles through which we read it today.

International developments pushed the change one step further. The Convention on the Rights of Persons with Disabilities does not stop at improving conditions of care; it asks whether the very structure of making decisions in a person's place remains justified. It shifts the starting point from 'What is good for this person?' to 'What does this person want, and how can we help them express and realize that will?' This is especially challenging in a field that includes acute psychosis, suicidality, and severe impairment of reality testing. Precisely because the question is difficult, it forces the system to distinguish diagnosis from incapacity, disagreement from dangerousness, and need for treatment from justification for deprivation of liberty.

One lesson repeated throughout the book is that diagnosis must never become a shortcut. A person does not lose their rights because a diagnosis has been entered in the medical record. Some people with severe mental disorders make complex decisions very well, while people without psychiatric diagnoses can be unable to decide during other medical conditions. The inquiry should be concrete: what does the person understand now, what is the risk, what do they want, what support could help them decide, and what is the least restrictive intervention capable of addressing the situation?

This also changes how coercion should be understood. Coercion is not only the decision made at the moment a door is locked. It is the result of a pathway. If a person could not obtain an appointment, if there was no crisis team in their area, if the family was left alone for days, and if the first available contact with the system was an overcrowded emergency department, the coercion seen at the end is not only a result of the person's mental condition. It is also a result of what was unavailable beforehand. Reducing coercion therefore cannot be achieved only by changing statutory language. It requires services that can be used before crisis reaches the edge.

Even inside a coercive event, autonomy remains in many areas. A person who cannot leave the ward may still be able to choose whom to speak with, what information may be shared with family, which medication they prefer, when to meet someone close to them, or what helps them calm down. A system that identifies the places where choice remains possible does not erase coercion, but it prevents coercion from spreading into every part of life. Deprivation of liberty in one domain is not permission to erase the person in every other domain.

The same principle applies to treatment without consent, restraint, and seclusion. Each adds a further interference and therefore requires its own justification. It is not enough to say that the person is already hospitalized involuntarily. The more invasive the intervention, the clearer the necessity, the more seriously alternatives must be examined, and the more carefully the decision must be documented for later review. Even when no alternative exists, the manner of intervention matters: language, privacy, explanation, and conversation after the event can affect trust and the willingness to seek help in the future.

The chapters on children, criminal law, and life after hospitalization showed that rights do not end at the hospital gate. A minor should participate in a way suited to age and understanding; a defendant with a mental disorder should be tried and treated without diagnosis erasing essential legal distinctions; and a person who has been discharged needs a genuine possibility of returning to work, housing, family, and community. If society continues to see the person first and foremost as 'mentally ill,' physical discharge remains incomplete.

This is also why the recovery model matters. The purpose of treatment is not merely to reduce symptoms but to make life possible. A person may continue to live with voices, anxiety, or fluctuations in mood and still work, love, study, and experience meaning. The system does not need to guarantee a life without difficulty; it needs to allow the person to build a life that is not defined only by difficulty. The shift in language may seem small, but it reverses priorities: treatment becomes a means to life, rather than life becoming a means to treatment.

The future of mental health care in Israel will probably not be a future without any coercion. Extreme situations will continue to place professionals and families before decisions in which no solution is perfect. But there is a great difference between a system in which coercion is a familiar tool used quickly and a system in which it is truly the last resort. Reaching the second system requires more than declarations of rights. It requires community services, emergency-hour availability, home treatment, crisis-respite houses, legal representation, advance directives, supported decision-making, and transparency mechanisms that allow the public to know where and how much force is being used.

The law will also have to adapt to such a system. The route may be comprehensive amendment of the current framework, or there may eventually be a place for new legislation. The name of the statute matters less than its starting point. Modern law should begin with the person and their rights, define the services and alternatives the state is obliged to develop, and only then specify the exceptional circumstances in which liberty may be restricted. That order is not merely aesthetic. It teaches the system what the rule is and what the exception is.

The final challenge is cultural. Even the best law cannot by itself create partnership if the professional who meets the patient sees primarily a risk. At the same time, a rights discourse that does not recognize the fear of families and the responsibility carried by staff will struggle to change reality. Genuine change requires more mutual trust: professionalism that is not afraid of review, law that respects clinical knowledge, families that receive support without becoming the owners of decision-making authority, and patients who are given a place not only as people telling their stories but as partners in designing services.

In the end, the movement from coercion toward autonomy is not a journey from one extreme to another. It is not a transition from a world in which people are treated to a world in which people merely choose. It is a change in the relationship between treatment and choice. The responsibility to protect a person does not disappear; it becomes more precise. It requires trying to preserve the person's life without turning that life into the property of the system.

And when that night comes again - when a person, a family, and a clinical team face a crisis without certainty - the question cannot be only whether it is lawful to take away liberty. We must also ask what was done to avoid reaching that point, what else can still be done now, who the person was before the crisis, what they would want if they could state it clearly, and how control will be returned as soon as the danger passes.

Perhaps this is the true test of a modern mental health system: not whether it knows how to use force when there is no alternative, but whether it knows how to build enough treatment, support, and trust around the person that the need for force becomes as rare as possible - and, when force is used, whether the system remembers that even in that moment the person before it does not stop having a life of their own, a voice of their own, and rights of their own.

Appendices

Appendix A

Key Timeline: Israel

1955 - Treatment of Mental Patients Law, 1955. The first Israeli statute to regulate psychiatric treatment and hospitalization comprehensively, including hospitalization without consent.

1991 - Mental Health Treatment Law, 1991. The new law replaced the 1955 statute and reorganized compulsory examination and hospitalization, psychiatric committees, court orders, and review procedures.

1992 - Basic Law: Human Dignity and Liberty. Established constitutional protection for life, bodily integrity, dignity, liberty, and privacy, and influenced the interpretation of legislation that interferes with liberty.

1996 - Patients' Rights Law, 1996. Entrenched, among other rights, the right to information, informed consent, privacy and confidentiality, and respect for patient dignity.

1998 - Equal Rights for Persons with Disabilities Law, 1998. Strengthened the shift from a model of charity to a model of equality, participation, and removal of barriers.

2000 - Community Rehabilitation of Persons with Mental Health Disabilities Law, 2000. Created a legal framework for community rehabilitation services. In 2024 the law's Hebrew name was amended to use the contemporary term for people living with mental health conditions.

2012 - Israel ratified the United Nations Convention on the Rights of Persons with Disabilities. The Convention added a significant international layer of equality, autonomy, and community living.

2015 - Implementation of the mental health insurance reform. Responsibility for providing mental health services within the national health basket was transferred to the health funds.

2016 - Amendment No. 18 to the Legal Capacity and Guardianship Law. Strengthened alternatives to guardianship and formally recognized supported decision-making.

2018 - Ministry of Health Director-General Circular 10/2018 on mechanical restraint and seclusion. Expressed an official policy of reducing restrictive measures and limiting their use to exceptional circumstances.

2024 - National Mental Health Program. Against the background of system needs and the effects of the Swords of Iron war, an additional annual budget of approximately NIS 1.4 billion was allocated and community responses were expanded.

2026 - Continued expansion of alternatives to hospitalization. The Ministry of Health describes crisis teams, ACT, day treatment, crisis-respite houses, and psychiatric home hospitalization as part of the public continuum of care; a government database updated to August 2026 lists dozens of supervised crisis-respite houses.

Appendix B

Key Timeline: The World

18th-19th centuries - Development of the asylum and 'moral treatment.' A gradual transition from conceptions of sin and exclusion toward medical and institutional frameworks.

1938 - Beginning of the use of electroconvulsive therapy (ECT). The treatment developed in Italy; its administration later changed substantially, and it remains an accepted medical treatment for certain conditions.

1950s - Beginning of the modern antipsychotic medication era. Chlorpromazine and other drugs made community treatment possible for some people and contributed to deinstitutionalization.

1961 - Erving Goffman published Asylums, an influential sociological critique of the 'total institution' and the loss of identity within institutional life.

1975 - O'Connor v. Donaldson. The U.S. Supreme Court held that mental illness alone does not justify confining a person who is not dangerous and can live safely in the community.

1978 - Italy's Law 180. The Basaglia reform marked a dramatic transition from traditional psychiatric hospitals toward community-based services.

1979 - Addington v. Texas. The U.S. Supreme Court required a heightened standard of proof in civil involuntary-commitment proceedings.

1979 - Winterwerp v. the Netherlands. The European Court of Human Rights articulated important conditions governing deprivation of liberty on the basis of mental disorder.

1983 - Mental Health Act in England and Wales. A central framework for involuntary hospitalization and treatment, subsequently amended and reformed over the years.

2006 - Adoption of the United Nations Convention on the Rights of Persons with Disabilities (CRPD). The Convention shifted the discourse toward equality, autonomy, equal recognition before the law, and community living.

2008 - The CRPD entered into force, beginning a significant period of interpretation, criticism, and legislative change in many countries.

2020 - The Dutch Wvggz entered into force. The new Dutch framework emphasizes compulsory treatment as a last resort and, in specified circumstances, permits compulsory treatment outside hospital.

2023 - OHCHR/WHO guidance on mental health legislation. Called for rights-based legislation, consent, community services, and reduction of coercion.

2025 - Mental Health Act 2025 in England and Wales. A major reform of the 1983 framework received Royal Assent; as of August 2026, most of the principal reforms were still scheduled for phased implementation.

Appendix C

Concise Glossary of Terms

Autonomy - A person's right and ability to make decisions concerning their life, body, and treatment in accordance with their values and preferences.

Involuntary hospitalization - Psychiatric hospitalization that is not based on the person's free consent and is carried out under legal authority.

Crisis-respite house - A relatively home-like community alternative to hospitalization that provides intensive care during a mental-health crisis for people who are suitable for the setting and consent to treatment.

Seclusion - Holding a patient alone in a designated space in a manner that restricts leaving it, in accordance with the applicable legal and professional framework.

De-escalation - Communication, environmental, and intervention strategies intended to reduce arousal, fear, or aggression and to prevent the need for physical force.

Deinstitutionalization - The process of reducing large psychiatric institutions and shifting the focus of treatment and rehabilitation to the community.

Recovery - An approach emphasizing a meaningful life, hope, choice, and participation in the community even when symptoms or limitations do not disappear completely.

Psychiatric advance directive - A document in which a person expresses in advance preferences concerning treatment and the management of a future crisis, for a period in which they may have difficulty expressing or making decisions.

Informed consent - Consent to treatment given after relevant information has been provided and understood, voluntarily and by a person who has the capacity to make the decision.

Mechanical restraint - Use of a physical device that restricts a patient's movement; an extreme measure subject to rules and oversight.

Psychiatric committee - A statutory body with review and decision-making functions concerning various matters related to involuntary hospitalization and treatment under Israeli law.

Covert coercion - Pressure that is not always imposed through a formal order or physical force but materially restricts a person's practical ability to refuse, for example an explicit or implied threat of increased restriction.

Decision-making capacity - The ability to understand relevant information, weigh it, and communicate a choice concerning a particular decision. Precise legal terminology varies among legal systems.

Dangerousness - An assessment of the risk of harm to oneself or others; it is not identical to the mere existence of a psychiatric diagnosis.

Least restrictive principle - The duty to prefer an intervention that achieves the required objective while interfering as little as possible with liberty and rights.

Peer specialist - A person with lived experience of mental-health challenges who participates in support, service delivery, training, or health-system planning.

District psychiatrist - A statutory office-holder in Israel's mental-health system who exercises powers under the Mental Health Treatment Law.

Supported decision-making - A mechanism in which a person makes decisions personally with assistance from another person, rather than transferring the decision entirely to someone else.

Community rehabilitation - A range of supports designed to enable participation in community life in areas such as housing, employment, education, social life, leisure, and other domains.

Crisis plan - A personal document identifying early warning signs, response strategies, contact persons, and treatment preferences for a future mental-health crisis.

Appendix D

Proposed Framework for Assessing Proportionality Before the Use of Coercion

The following framework is not draft legislation and is not a substitute for professional judgment. It is offered as a structured tool for decision-making:

1. What is the current clinical condition? Describe facts and symptoms, not diagnosis alone.
2. What is the anticipated risk or harm? Define to whom, at what level of severity, and within what time frame.
3. What is the factual basis for the risk assessment? Behavior, statements, history, and other relevant information.
4. What is the person's capacity to make the specific decision? Do not infer incapacity merely from refusal.
5. What support has been provided to enable decision-making? Explanation, time, a trusted supporter, interpretation, or other accommodations.
6. What does the person want, and what are they afraid of? Document the person's position even when it is not accepted.
7. What less restrictive alternatives are available? Community care, home treatment, day treatment, a crisis-respite house, voluntary hospitalization, or other measures.
8. Why are those alternatives insufficient in this case? Provide an individualized explanation rather than a general formula.
9. What is the minimum duration of intervention required? Set a clear point for reassessment.
10. What harm might coercion itself cause? Trauma, loss of trust, adverse effects, and impaired functioning.

11. Who will review the decision, and when? Professional review, a psychiatric committee, or a court, as applicable.
12. What is the plan for ending coercion? From the moment coercion begins, consider how and when it can be reduced and discontinued.

Appendix E

Selected Foundational Sources

Methodological Note, Sources, and Edition Update

This book is an interdisciplinary research-based work of nonfiction combining history, law, health policy, ethics, and mental-health scholarship. This appendix brings together the foundational sources on which the discussion rests and enables readers to locate the legal and research basis of the book's principal claims without interrupting the flow of the main text.

Major legislation, regulations, procedures, and official documents were checked against the governmental legal and information databases available through August 22, 2026. Where a description in this book conflicts with the binding text of current law or an updated official document, the official and current text governs. Case law, legislation, and administrative procedures may change after the edition's closing date.

The research bibliography uses a consistent format including author, year, title, journal or publisher, volume and pages, and DOI where available. Sources were selected because of their status as primary sources, foundational works, systematic reviews, or major publications in the fields discussed.

Israeli Legislation and Regulations

- Treatment of Mentally Ill Persons Law, 1955 (repealed when the 1991 law entered into force).
- Mental Health Treatment Law, 1991, as amended; National Legislation Database, the Knesset.
- Mental Health Treatment Regulations, 1992, as amended.
- Mental Health Treatment Regulations (Legal Representation in Compulsory Treatment), 2006.

- Patients' Rights Law, 1996, as amended.
- Equal Rights for Persons with Disabilities Law, 1998, as amended.
- Community Rehabilitation of Persons with Mental Health Disabilities Law, 2000 (under its updated Hebrew name following Amendment No. 2, 2024).
- Legal Capacity and Guardianship Law, 1962, especially Amendment No. 18, 2016, concerning supported decision-making and alternatives to guardianship.

Official Documents, Data, and Policy in Israel

- Ministry of Health. Involuntary psychiatric hospitalization and treatment of adults. Official public information concerning the grounds for coercion, authorized decision-makers, periods of hospitalization, extensions, appeals, and legal representation.
- Ministry of Health, Director-General Circular 10/2018, Mechanical Restraint and Seclusion of Patients in Psychiatric Hospitalization, April 1, 2018.
- Ministry of Health. Guide to the Rights of Persons Hospitalized in the Psychiatric System, current version.
- Ministry of Health. Official information on compulsory outpatient psychiatric treatment, open and locked wards, psychiatric home hospitalization, crisis-respite houses, day treatment, and crisis teams.
- Ministry of Health. Mental-health statistical yearbooks and government databases concerning hospitalization, community care, workforce, and services.
- State Comptroller of Israel. Audit reports concerning involuntary psychiatric hospitalization and treatment, community mental-health services, workforce, and conditions of hospitalization.
- Knesset Research and Information Center. Background papers and reviews concerning the mental-health system, hospitalization, rehabilitation, and reforms.

- Bank of Israel. Annual Report 2025, including discussion of the mental-health system from the 2015 reform through the effects of the war and the growth in demand for services.

Selected Israeli Case Law

- Leave for Civil Appeal 8000/07, Attorney General v. Anonymous (Supreme Court of Israel, May 2, 2012) - authority of the psychiatric committee to extend involuntary hospitalization, evidentiary basis, proportionality, and consideration of less restrictive alternatives.
- Leave for Civil Appeal 2967/16, Anonymous v. District Psychiatric Committee et al. (Supreme Court of Israel, April 14, 2016) - judicial review of an extension of involuntary hospitalization and the need for an individualized and current assessment.
- Decisions of Israeli district courts and the Supreme Court concerning psychiatric committees, dangerousness, liberty, legal representation, compulsory outpatient treatment, and application of proportionality, as discussed in the relevant chapters.

International Law and Human Rights

- United Nations. (2006). Convention on the Rights of Persons with Disabilities (CRPD).
- Committee on the Rights of Persons with Disabilities. (2014). General Comment No. 1: Article 12 - Equal Recognition before the Law, CRPD/C/GC/1.
- Committee on the Rights of Persons with Disabilities. (2015). Guidelines on Article 14 of the Convention: The Right to Liberty and Security of Persons with Disabilities.
- World Health Organization & Office of the United Nations High Commissioner for Human Rights. (2023). Mental Health, Human Rights and Legislation: Guidance and Practice. Geneva: WHO & OHCHR. ISBN 978-92-4-008073-7; HR/PUB/23/3.

- Council of Europe. European Convention on Human Rights, Article 5.
- United Kingdom. Mental Health Act 1983, as amended; Mental Health Act 2025.
- United Kingdom. Mental Capacity Act 2005.
- Netherlands. Wet verplichte geestelijke gezondheidszorg (Wvggz), Act of 24 January 2018, in force from 1 January 2020, as amended.

Selected International Case Law

- O'Connor v. Donaldson, 422 U.S. 563 (1975).
- Addington v. Texas, 441 U.S. 418 (1979).
- Winterwerp v. the Netherlands, App. No. 6301/73, European Court of Human Rights, 24 October 1979.
- H.L. v. the United Kingdom, App. No. 45508/99, European Court of Human Rights, 5 October 2004.
- Stanev v. Bulgaria [GC], App. No. 36760/06, European Court of Human Rights, 17 January 2012.
- Rooman v. Belgium [GC], App. No. 18052/11, European Court of Human Rights, 31 January 2019.

Historical, Sociological, and Critical Literature

- Goffman, E. (1961). Asylums: Essays on the Social Situation of Mental Patients and Other Inmates. Garden City, NY: Anchor Books.
- Foucault, M. (2006). History of Madness. J. Murphy & J. Khalfa (Trans.). London: Routledge. (Original work published 1961).
- Szasz, T. S. (1961). The Myth of Mental Illness: Foundations of a Theory of Personal Conduct. New York: Harper & Row.
- Laing, R. D. (1960). The Divided Self: An Existential Study in Sanity and Madness. London: Tavistock.

The historical critical sources are presented in this book as influential intellectual traditions, not as substitutes for contemporary clinical knowledge. Where historiographical or medical disagreement exists, the book distinguishes their contribution to public and professional discourse from current scientific consensus.

Recovery, Community Care, and Deinstitutionalization

- Anthony, W. A. (1993). Recovery from mental illness: The guiding vision of the mental health service system in the 1990s. Psychosocial Rehabilitation Journal, 16(4), 11-23. doi:10.1037/h0095655.
- Thornicroft, G., & Tansella, M. (2013). The balanced care model: The case for both hospital- and community-based mental healthcare. British Journal of Psychiatry, 202(4), 246-248. doi:10.1192/bjp.bp.112.111377.
- Seikkula, J., Aaltonen, J., Alakare, B., Haarakangas, K., Keränen, J., & Lehtinen, K. (2006). Five-year experience of first-episode nonaffective psychosis in open-dialogue approach: Treatment principles, follow-up outcomes, and two case studies. Psychotherapy Research, 16(2), 214-228.
- World Health Organization. (2021). Guidance on Community Mental Health Services: Promoting Person-Centred and Rights-Based Approaches. Geneva: WHO.

Autonomy, Supported Decision-Making, and Advance Directives

- Pathare, S., & Shields, L. S. (2012). Supported decision-making for persons with mental illness: A review. Public Health Reviews, 34, Article 15. doi:10.1007/BF03391683.
- Penzenstadler, L., Molodynski, A., & Khazaal, Y. (2020). Supported decision making for people with mental health disorders in clinical practice: A systematic review.

International Journal of Psychiatry in Clinical Practice, 24(1), 3-9. doi:10.1080/13651501.2019.1676452.

- Francis, C. J., Hazelton, M., & Wilson, R. L. (2024). Supported decision-making interventions in mental healthcare: A systematic review. Health Expectations, 27(6), e70134. doi:10.1111/hex.70134.
- Szmukler, G., Daw, R., & Callard, F. (2014). Mental health law and the UN Convention on the Rights of Persons with Disabilities. International Journal of Law and Psychiatry, 37(3), 245-252. doi:10.1016/j.ijlp.2013.11.024.
- Swanson, J. W., Swartz, M. S., et al. (2006). Psychiatric advance directives among public mental health consumers in five U.S. cities: Prevalence, demand, and correlates. Journal of the American Academy of Psychiatry and the Law, 34(1), 43-57.
- Swanson, J. W., Swartz, M. S., et al. (2006). Superseding psychiatric advance directives: Ethical and legal considerations. Journal of the American Academy of Psychiatry and the Law, 34(3), 385-394.

Coercion, Restraint, Seclusion, and Reduction of Restrictive Measures

- Chieze, M., Hurst, S., Kaiser, S., & Sentissi, O. (2019). Effects of seclusion and restraint in adult psychiatry: A systematic review. Frontiers in Psychiatry, 10, 491. doi:10.3389/fpsyt.2019.00491.
- Goulet, M.-H., Larue, C., & Dumais, A. (2017). Evaluation of seclusion and restraint reduction programs in mental health: A systematic review. Aggression and Violent Behavior, 34, 139-146. doi:10.1016/j.avb.2017.01.019.
- World Health Organization & OHCHR. (2023). Mental Health, Human Rights and Legislation: Guidance and Practice, sections addressing free and informed consent, involuntary detention, seclusion, restraint, and alternatives to coercion.

- Ministry of Health, Director-General Circular 10/2018 - the principal normative-professional source used in this book for the discussion of mechanical restraint and seclusion in Israeli psychiatric inpatient care.

The Least Restrictive Principle

The discussion in this book of proportionality, alternatives to hospitalization, and renewed review of continuing coercion draws cumulatively on Basic Law: Human Dignity and Liberty and the Mental Health Treatment Law.

References by the Book's Main Lines of Discussion

Parts One-Three: The Birth of Institutional Psychiatry, the Era of Coercion, and the Transition to Rights.

Principal sources: Goffman; Foucault; Szasz; Laing; O'Connor v. Donaldson; Addington v. Texas; Winterwerp v. the Netherlands; historical literature on deinstitutionalization and civil rights.

Part Four: Israel - From the Early State to the Mental Health Treatment Law.

Treatment of Mentally Ill Persons Law, 1955; Mental Health Treatment Law, 1991; 1992 Regulations; National Legislation Database; documents of the Knesset and Ministry of Health.

Part Five: The Rights Revolution in Israel.

Basic Law: Human Dignity and Liberty; Patients' Rights Law; Equal Rights for Persons with Disabilities Law; Community Rehabilitation of Persons with Mental Health Disabilities Law; Amendment No. 18 to the Legal Capacity and Guardianship Law.

Part Six: Reform, Recovery, and Supported Decision-Making.

Ministry of Health materials on the reform and community services; Anthony; Thornicroft & Tansella; Pathare & Shields;

Penzenstadler et al.; Francis et al.; Swanson et al.; WHO community mental-health guidance.

Part Seven: Coercion Under the Test of Human Rights.

Mental Health Treatment Law and Regulations; Ministry of Health materials on involuntary hospitalization; Director-General Circular 10/2018; Leave for Civil Appeal 8000/07; Leave for Civil Appeal 2967/16; Chieze et al.; Goulet et al.; WHO/OHCHR 2023.

Part Eight: Children, Criminal Law, and Life After Hospitalization.

Relevant provisions of the Mental Health Treatment Law and criminal law; Ministry of Health documents; literature on recovery, community care, continuity of care, and rights.

Part Nine: The New International Revolution.

CRPD; General Comment No. 1; Committee guidance concerning Article 14; WHO/OHCHR 2023; European Convention on Human Rights; Mental Health Act 1983 and Mental Health Act 2025; Mental Capacity Act 2005; Wvggz; ECtHR case law.

Part Ten: Israel Put to the Test and the Reform Proposal.

Mental Health Treatment Law in its current version; Israeli rights legislation; State Comptroller reports; Ministry of Health and Knesset documents; Bank of Israel; CRPD; WHO/OHCHR; Szmukler et al.; literature on least restrictive measures, decision-making capacity, and reduction of coercion.

Principles for Evaluating Claims and Sources

When using this book academically, readers are encouraged to distinguish among four categories of source: binding law - legislation and case law; institutional documents - procedures, circulars, and reports; research literature - empirical studies and reviews; and interpretive literature - history, criticism, and theory. This distinction helps prevent critical literature from being treated as clinical data, or a policy guideline from being treated as law.

In chapters dealing with comparative law, the purpose of comparison is to illuminate models and principles, not to suggest that foreign law applies in Israel. Any specific legal analysis should consult the current text of the law and case law in the relevant jurisdiction.

In chapters dealing with coercion, restraint, and seclusion, research findings should be read together with their methodological limitations. The book does not present complex associations as certain causation where the literature does not support such a conclusion.

Bibliographic Consistency

Journal and book titles are presented in English in their original language; Israeli laws and documents are identified by their official Hebrew titles in the Hebrew edition and by consistent English renderings in this English edition. DOI information is included where available and checked. Dates for governmental internet sources refer to the version available when this edition was closed.

Recommended Supplementary Sources

- World Health Organization. QualityRights materials and tools on mental health, recovery, community inclusion, and human rights.
- World Health Organization. (2021). Guidance and Technical Packages on Community Mental Health Services: Promoting Person-Centred and Rights-Based Approaches.
- United Nations Office of the High Commissioner for Human Rights. Materials concerning the CRPD, legal capacity, liberty and security, and participation of persons with psychosocial disabilities.
- Ministry of Health - the Hebrew-language “Healthy Mind” (Benefesh Bria) website: current information on rights, psychiatric hospitalization, community services, alternatives to hospitalization, and rehabilitation.

- Knesset National Legislation Database - official texts, amendments, and secondary legislation concerning the Mental Health Treatment Law and related statutes.
- Israel Judicial Authority and legal case-law databases - full texts of judgments and case-law updates.

Closing Academic Note

The references and bibliography in this appendix are intended to make the book's discussion transparent, verifiable, and open to further study without changing its character as accessible research-based nonfiction. They complement the explanations in the body of the book and clarify the normative, institutional, and research foundation of each major line of discussion.

In preparation for the closing of this edition in August 2026, the principal legal sources and official documents underlying the chapters on law, involuntary hospitalization, restrictive measures, and international comparison were rechecked. Major research sources were standardized bibliographically, and DOI information was included where available.

This book is not a substitute for individualized medical or legal advice. Its research purpose is to analyze development, compare models, and propose a source-based framework for discussing the balance between treatment and protection, on the one hand, and liberty, autonomy, and human dignity, on the other.

www.ingramcontent.com/pod-product-compliance
Lightning Source LLC
LaVergne TN
LVHW010714061126
851857LV00014B/1175
9789659339747

addressing problems quickly. The absence of effective governance creates environments where problems can escalate unchecked.

Finally, digital transformation must be viewed as an ongoing journey rather than a destination. Organizations that treat transformation as a one-time project often struggle to adapt to changing circumstances and miss opportunities for continuous improvement. Building organizational capabilities for ongoing innovation and adaptation is more important than any specific technology implementation.

The Integration of AI and Future Technologies

As we look toward the future of digital transformation, artificial intelligence will play an increasingly central role in how organizations operate and compete. However, the integration of AI into business operations requires careful consideration of both opportunities and limitations.

Current AI implementations in ERP systems often fall short of vendor promises, focusing on narrow, specific use cases rather than the transformational capabilities that are often marketed. Organizations must approach AI with realistic expectations while building the foundational data quality and analytical capabilities necessary for future success.

The key to successful AI implementation lies not in the sophistication of the algorithms themselves, but in the organization's ability to integrate AI insights into decision-making processes and business workflows. This requires not only technical infrastructure but also cultural change, process redesign, and workforce development.

As AI capabilities continue to evolve, organizations must develop frameworks for evaluating and implementing new technologies based on genuine business value rather than technological novelty. This includes establishing ethical guidelines for AI use, ensuring transparency in automated decision-making, and maintaining human oversight of critical business processes.

Final Thoughts: The Path to Digital Excellence

As businesses and organizations continue their digital journeys, the fundamental question remains: How will they navigate the complexities of the digital jungle while avoiding the pitfalls that have trapped so many others? The answer lies in embracing change with strategic purpose, leveraging technology intelligently, and cultivating leadership capabilities that can thrive in uncertainty.

The digital age is not about merely surviving—it is about thriving. Organizations that master digital transformation with foresight, flexibility, and firm leadership will not only stay competitive but will redefine industries, create new opportunities, and build a future where innovation and efficiency drive sustainable growth.

The lessons learned from both spectacular failures and remarkable successes provide a roadmap for navigating digital transformation successfully. Organizations must approach transformation with humility, learning from the mistakes of others while building on proven success patterns. This requires honest assessment of organizational readiness, realistic expectation setting, and unwavering commitment to the cultural and operational changes necessary for sustainable success.

The journey through the digital jungle is challenging, but the rewards are vast for those who dare to lead with wisdom gained from experience. As the digital landscape continues to evolve, those who remain agile, data-driven, and visionary will be the ones who shape the future rather than simply react to it.

Success in digital transformation is not guaranteed by technology adoption alone—it requires strategic thinking, cultural transformation, and operational excellence executed with persistence and adaptability. The organizations that master these dimensions will not only survive the digital jungle but will emerge as leaders capable of creating the next wave of innovation and transformation.

Welcome to the digital age—where mastering the jungle requires learning from both triumph and failure, maintaining strategic focus amid complexity, and never losing sight of the human dimensions that ultimately determine success or failure. The question is not whether digital transformation is necessary, but how effectively it can be executed with wisdom gained from those who have traveled this path before.

The future belongs to organizations that approach digital transformation as both a technological and human journey, combining cutting-edge capabilities with timeless principles of leadership, communication, and change management. In this synthesis of innovation and wisdom lies the key to not just surviving but mastering the digital jungle.

About the Author

Eric Kimberling is the CEO and Founder of Third Stage Consulting Group, a leading independent advisory firm specializing in digital transformation and enterprise technology selection, and Chairman of Lander Talent. With over 20 years of experience in organizational change and technology implementation, Kimberling has guided hundreds of organizations through complex ERP selections, system implementations, and digital transformation initiatives.

As a recognized thought leader in the enterprise software industry, Kimberling has helped organizations across diverse sectors—from Fortune 500 companies to mid-market businesses and government agencies—navigate the critical decisions that determine the success or failure of their technology investments. His expertise spans strategic planning, vendor selection, risk mitigation, and change management for large-scale digital initiatives.

Kimberling is a frequent keynote speaker at industry conferences and has authored numerous articles and research studies on digital transformation best practices. His insights have been featured in leading business publications, and he regularly provides commentary on emerging trends in enterprise technology and organizational change management.

Through Third Stage Consulting Group, Kimberling has witnessed firsthand both the spectacular successes and costly failures that define the digital transformation landscape. This unique vantage point—working as an independent advisor rather than a vendor or systems integrator—has provided him with unbiased insights into what drives transformation success and failure across different industries and organizational contexts.

His practical, results-oriented approach combines strategic thinking with real-world experience, making him a trusted advisor to executives seeking to maximize their return on digital transformation investments while minimizing the risks that have derailed so many well-intentioned initiatives.

www.ingramcontent.com/pod-product-compliance
Lightning Source LLC
LaVergne TN
LVHW010710061126
851857LV00014B/1119
* 9 7 9 8 2 3 4 1 7 4 6 4 2 *